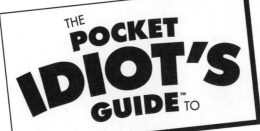

THE POCKET IDIOT'S GUIDE TO

Great Buns and Thighs

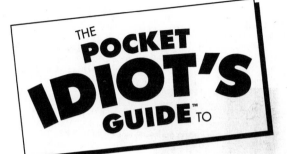

THE POCKET IDIOT'S GUIDE™ TO

Great Buns and Thighs

by Tom Seabourne

ALPHA

A member of the Penguin Group (USA) Inc.

ALPHA BOOKS

Published by the Penguin Group

Penguin Group (USA) Inc., 375 Hudson Street, New York, New York 10014, U.S.A.

Penguin Group (Canada), 10 Alcorn Avenue, Toronto, Ontario, Canada M4V 3B2 (a division of Pearson Penguin Canada Inc.)

Penguin Books Ltd, 80 Strand, London WC2R 0RL, England

Penguin Ireland, 25 St Stephen's Green, Dublin 2, Ireland (a division of Penguin Books Ltd)

Penguin Group (Australia), 250 Camberwell Road, Camberwell, Victoria 3124, Australia (a division of Pearson Australia Group Pty Ltd)

Penguin Books India Pvt Ltd, 11 Community Centre, Panchsheel Park, New Delhi—110 017, India

Penguin Group (NZ), cnr Airborne and Rosedale Roads, Albany, Auckland 1310, New Zealand (a division of Pearson New Zealand Ltd)

Penguin Books (South Africa) (Pty) Ltd, 24 Sturdee Avenue, Rosebank, Johannesburg 2196, South Africa

Penguin Books Ltd, Registered Offices: 80 Strand, London WC2R 0RL, England

International Standard Book Number: 1-59257-443-2
Library of Congress Catalog Card Number: 2005932771

07 06 05   8 7 6 5 4 3 2 1

Interpretation of the printing code: The rightmost number of the first series of numbers is the year of the book's printing; the rightmost number of the second series of numbers is the number of the book's printing. For example, a printing code of 05-1 shows that the first printing occurred in 2005.

Printed in the United States of America

Note: This publication contains the opinions and ideas of its author. It is intended to provide helpful and informative material on the subject matter covered. It is sold with the understanding that the author and publisher are not engaged in rendering professional services in the book. If the reader requires personal assistance or advice, a competent professional should be consulted.

The author and publisher specifically disclaim any responsibility for any liability, loss, or risk, personal or otherwise, which is incurred as a consequence, directly or indirectly, of the use and application of any of the contents of this book.

Most Alpha books are available at special quantity discounts for bulk purchases for sales promotions, premiums, fund-raising, or educational use. Special books, or book excerpts, can also be created to fit specific needs.

For details, write: Special Markets, Alpha Books, 375 Hudson Street, New York, NY 10014.

This book is dedicated to my wife, Danese.

Contents

Appendix

Introduction

Caboose, hiney. It doesn't matter what you want to call it, your buns are your largest and most attractive muscle group in your body. Your thighs are good-looking, too, but your buns get the vote for the sexiest body part by both men and women. A firm, lifted set of glutes is appealing to everyone, and you look better in your clothes, too. With a slim waistline and firm, well-shaped buns, you have a better hourglass shape, allowing skirts and pants to fit better. Cultures around the world define attractive women as having a beautiful butt. And women prefer men with muscular legs and tight glutes.

However, women often obsess about the dreaded "saddlebags" and men worry about needing a "butt-lift." This is a complete program of motivation, diet, and butt-sculpting exercise. This three-pronged approach gives you all of the ammo you need to attack your problem areas on all fronts.

Maybe you had trouble staying on a program in the past, but we guarantee that our workout is do-able. You have the desire because you picked up this book. Now make the commitment. We shower you with motivational tips until your workouts become habit. In a week you will notice muscles that you didn't know existed. And when you see sculpted thighs and buns in the mirror, you will be hooked.

There is no way to spot-reduce fat around your hips and thighs, but if you eat right you will be able to uncover those firm, sexy glutes. Eating correctly is easier than you think. You may not be eating enough. Or maybe you should eat more meals each day. We take the guesswork out of starving cellulite. Our eating program whittles away cellulite until it becomes microscopic.

Rhythmic exercises burn the fat that surrounds your toned thighs and buns. As the term implies, rhythmic activities are smooth, steady, easy movements that you can do indoors or out, depending on your mood and the weather. For example, you can walk, pedal, step, dance, roll, or slide. We have so many rhythmic activities to choose from that you will never become bored.

Most people don't want their butts and thighs to grow bigger, but they wouldn't mind toning them. We teach you to firm your butt and thighs without putting on unwanted weight. Small changes in the way you move stimulate flabby muscles. Muscles need to be activated in order for them to tone up. Stimulating muscle firms it and gives you the shape that you have been dreaming about.

Women prefer having thighs and a tight butt with good definition. Definition refers to that dimple on the side of the hip. Naysayers believe that a good-looking, chiseled set of glutes is in the genes, so to speak. But you can drastically improve your shape using isolation exercises. Many people have never set foot inside a gym but have learned to incorporate our thigh- and butt-shaping isolation exercises into their daily routine. Every well-planned move you make can train your butt and thigh muscles.

You can do these moves at home or at work without expensive equipment.

You may decide to increase your intensity by heading to the gym. The hard part about training the butt and thighs in the gym is to do the exercises correctly. We tweak your training program so that you are targeting your glutes and thighs at every angle. Simple changes in position, posture, and weight distribution have a dramatic effect on achieving the well-shaped set of glutes and thighs you desire.

You may decide to cross-train with our other two books, *The Pocket Idiot's Guide to a Great Upper Body* and *The Pocket Idiot's Guide to Great Abs*. Practice the strategies in these three programs and we can't wait to see the new you.

The purpose of this book is not to turn you into an exercise fanatic or health-food nut. There is no need to do squats hours a day or to eat perfectly. Exercise a little each day and eat right most of the time.

In this book you will find sidebars that are tidbits of important and useful information to keep you making progress on the program.

Bet You Didn't Know

This sidebar warns you of common myths and misconceptions concerning diet and exercise.

Get It Right

This sidebar provides you with cautionary warnings to be sure you're doing your exercises right.

In Other Words

This sidebar helps you to understand the anatomy of your buns and thighs and figure out technical or unusual terms and concepts found in the main text. For example, gluteus medius, quadriceps, vastus lateralis.

Your Personal Trainer

This sidebar provides you with quick tips about how to do your exercises correctly and information to keep your form perfect.

Acknowledgments

I want to thank the photographer, Ron Barker, and our fabulous models, Brittany and Brandon. Thanks to Paul Dinas, who had the confidence in me to pursue this project, and his amazing coaching along the way. My wife, Danese, and five beautiful children, Alaina, Grant, Laura, Susanna, and Julia, are always finding new ways to make workouts fun. And finally to my brother, Rick, my sister, Barb, and my mother, Ann, who, in my opinion, own the finest fitness facility in northeastern Pennsylvania.

Special Thanks to the Technical Reviewer

The Pocket Idiot's Guide to Great Buns and Thighs was reviewed by an expert who double-checked the accuracy of what you'll learn here, to help us ensure that this book gives you everything you need to know. Special thanks are extended to Shannon Loveless.

Trademarks

All terms mentioned in this book that are known to be or are suspected of being trademarks or service marks have been appropriately capitalized. Alpha Books and Penguin Group (USA) Inc. cannot attest to the accuracy of this information. Use of a term in this book should not be regarded as affecting the validity of any trademark or service mark.

Chapter 1

Body Made Simple: Buns and Thighs

In This Chapter

- Thinner thighs and glamorous glutes can be yours
- Define your legs your way
- The body you want, bottoms-up

The perfect body is an "X" shape. The top of the X is your shoulders and upper back, narrowing into your waist and hips. The bottom of the X is long legs with upper thighs that appear to connect directly to the waist. The legs are the most important part to develop. When trained correctly, they make your waist look smaller and complete the X shape.

Everyone loves a nice pair of legs. What you do with them, however, will greatly affect how they look. The hips, butt, and thighs are the problem areas, where women accumulate most of their cellulite. Unfortunately, for women nature has designated fat cells in the lower body to serve as energy storage for pregnancy and lactation.

Men generally store most of their fat in their bellies. They try to build up their chests and arms to compensate. But nothing looks more ridiculous than a guy whose arms are bigger than his legs.

Many women fear they will get bulky legs if they lift weights, but you won't get "bulky" if you train correctly. You may actually lose size by lifting weights because you become more compact. When training, it's important not only to know where your muscles are, but also what they do so you can sculpt them accordingly. Here's a brief overview of the lower-body muscles.

In Other Words

Fast-twitch, type IIB fibers are white, powerful, and larger than the slow-twitch, type I, red endurance fibers.

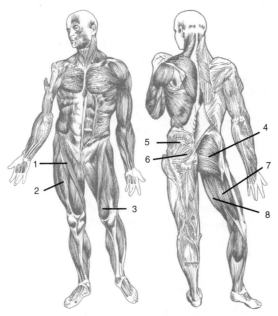

1. Adductors (inner upper thighs)
2. Rectus femoris (middle thigh)
3. Vastus medialis (inner lower thigh)
4. Gluteus maximus (backside)
5. Gluteus minimus (side of butt - inner)
6. Gluteus medius (side of butt - outer)
7. Biceps femoris (middle hamstrings)
8. Semitendinosus (inner hamstrings)

Buns and thighs diagram.

Thighs

Female fashion models are tall with very long legs. Believe it or not, some people are born this way!

Others, unfortunately, are somewhere on the continuum between "model" legs and thick, short, stubby legs. If you weren't born with the genetics of a model, you can get closer to the long-legged look by weight training.

If you have decent leg development in proportion to the rest of your body, you'll look sexy. And although your thigh muscles require intense workouts to see results, your goal is to keep your whole body in proportion.

Train your entire thigh from top to bottom. Check out people at the beach and you will see "carrot thighs"—big on top and in the middle, but no development in the lower thigh. A well-shaped thigh should be nearly as wide at the bottom part as at the mid part. Carrot-shaped legs can throw off your symmetry. A good thigh sweep will offset a thick waist. In bodybuilding, the "sweep" refers to the symmetrical development of the outer thigh muscle (vastus lateralis) and the lower part of the hourglass shape—the larger the chest and back and the larger the hips and thigh sweep, the smaller the waistline appears. The *quads* are the front part of the thighs, and as the name implies, consist of four muscles. The *rectus femoris*, the large muscle in the center of the thigh, crosses both the knee and hip. It connects from your pelvis to below the kneecap. This muscle can help you bend your hip or straighten your knee.

The *vastus lateralis* is your very visible outer thigh muscle. This muscle provides the "sweep"—the lower part of the "X" that creates the illusion that your legs attach directly to your waist. When you have well-defined legs, there is a perceptible separation between this muscle and the hamstrings muscle in the back of your legs. A good thigh sweep will offset a thick waist.

Your *vastus medialis* is on the inside of your thigh. It creates that "teardrop" appearance just above the knee. Keep this muscle strong to prevent knee problems and to balance out your entire set of thigh muscles.

The *vastus intermedius*, underneath the rectus femoris, runs from the top of the thighbone to the knee and works to straighten the knee. Place your right hand on your right thigh. Extend your right foot out in front. You can feel the vastus intermedius and your other thigh muscles flexing. These large muscles can be compared to the muscle on the back of your upper arm. That is, by flexing, they straighten the leg.

Different foot positioning during leg exercises targets different areas of the thighs. For greater overall development of the front thigh, keep your toes pointed forward and have your feet just outside your shoulders. Pointing the toes out with a wide stance targets the glutes as well. To firm your inner thighs, point your toes out but keep your feet closer. For outer thigh development (the sweep), keep your legs close and toes pointed straight ahead.

Heavy squats and partial range of motion leg presses develop the upper thigh, hips, and butt. The teardrop-shaped lower-thigh muscle can be developed with a narrower stance. The front squat shapes the upper thigh because it targets your rectus femoris, which goes all the way up to your hips. When this muscle is developed, it makes your legs appear longer.

Get It Right

Balancing the size and strength between your thighs and hamstrings not only keeps your legs looking great, but it protects the stability of your knees.

Hamstrings

In gyms you may notice lines of people waiting at the bench press while the hamstrings machine sits idle. Many males who work out to build size are concerned with getting their chests huge and biceps bulging, and often place too much emphasis on their arm workouts while neglecting to do anything for their hamstrings. What they may not realize is that if they train their legs, the muscles of the upper body are stimulated, too.

To get defined arms, you work your biceps. Your hamstrings are considered your leg-biceps. A thick, rounded set of hamstrings are muscles that stand out.

Women have a different reason to train their hamstrings—cellulite. Every woman has cellulite. Cellulite is simply fat, water, and toxins under the tissue beneath the skin, causing that "cottage cheese" appearance.

Whether you want to build muscle, lose fat, or incinerate cellulite, your hamstrings workout is a huge part of the solution. Legs, as a whole, are neglected, but the hamstrings are the forlorn stepchildren. The hamstrings lie along the length of rear thigh. They connect near the butt and the back of the knee. Leg flexing or bending uses the hamstrings muscles. They act in the same manner as the front of your arm (ergo leg-biceps).

The three muscles of your hamstrings are the *biceps femoris*, *semitendinosus*, and *semimembranosus*.

The bicep femoris (leg biceps) is the outer sweep of the hamstring. When you turn sideways, this is the muscle that gives your leg that full, sexy look. It has two heads; the long head crosses the knee and the hip, the short one only crosses the knee. These muscles curl the lower leg up toward your butt, and work with your butt muscles to straighten your hip.

As much as you may hate training your hamstrings, it is the most impressive part of your upper leg. Nothing looks better than seeing a firm, rounded group of hamstrings muscles. To improve the lines and symmetry in your hamstrings, train with enough weight that the tenth repetition is a challenge. Your hamstrings are mostly fast-twitch muscle fibers.

If you want your hamstrings to be round and full, train them by doing leg curls. The secret to filling out your hamstring muscle is to keep your ankles relaxed. If you flex your ankle, you use your calf muscle in your lower leg to do the work that the hamstrings are supposed to do.

Train your hamstrings at different angles and intensities to get full development. You can vary your toe position when doing exercises to target different areas of your hamstrings. When you add density to your hamstrings you create a perfect balance with your thighs.

Your Personal Trainer _____

Firm those buns all day long. Whenever you are about to sit, stand, stoop, or bend down, lead with your buns and keep your back straight.

Buns

If you were born with a round bottom, you lucked out. If you don't have buns of steel, you are not alone. Stand up and take a good look at your butt. You probably think that it is too small, too saggy, too flabby, or too big. Maintaining your shapely buns is a fight against gravity. Owning a great set of buns is hot, but cellulite is not. Imagine cellulite on the outside of your butt as a wrinkled-up, old balloon. Your butt muscles are the air in the balloon. If you blow up the rubber balloon by firming up your muscles, the wrinkles go away and the rubber on the balloon gets thinner.

While aerobic exercise burns calories, lower-body resistance training is a quick way to tone muscle and help reduce cellulite. By firming the butt muscles below the fat, the cellulite on top of the muscle thins out.

The *gluteus maximus* (butt muscle) is the largest and most superficial of the three buttocks muscles that form the gluteal complex. So that's where most of your firming will take place. The glutes originates on the back of your pelvis and attaches to the rear thighbone. The glutes are the muscles responsible for moving your legs backward and outward. They are the most powerful muscles in the body. You use your gluteals whenever you step, sit, or stand. While standing, place your right hand on your right bun and raise your right leg backward a couple of inches off of the floor. Feel your glutes flex? This is the muscle that gives your butt that lifted look.

Straightening your legs from a bent-knee position requires you to straighten your hip. This is a major function of your glutes. Stand up from your chair and you will feel your glutes tighten. If you want to really activate your glutes, press through your heels when you stand up. You just performed the up phase of a squat called hip extension.

Unlike muscles such as the thigh, the glutes are nearly impossible to train by themselves. When you train your thighs or hamstrings, your glutes usually help. Since butt firming and toning is a side effect of training your legs, you may not have to give them a second thought.

Even without butt-specific training, you may already have firm tight buns from everything else you do. But if you don't have the firm butt you desire, small adjustments in your leg workouts can maximize your maximus.

> **Bet You Didn't Know**
>
> Lifting weights tightens, trims, and firms muscle. And no worries of developing a big butt. If you train properly, you can actually lose inches. Women are generally stronger in their lower body than in their upper body, so they should make sure to train with lower weights/high reps. This will keep them from building too much muscle, and keep their body in proportion.

You can maximize gluteal stimulation during the squat by adopting a wider stance. From a wide stance, you increase hip extension and decrease knee extension, so the emphasis shifts somewhat from your thighs to your glutes.

Outer Hips

Some people gain cellulite in their lower body while others gain fat around their midsection. You have probably heard about pear-shaped and apple-shaped body types, but there is more to your anatomical structure than just fat deposits.

If you have trouble with your saddlebags, flat fanny, thunder-thighs, or bubble buns, change your silhouette by training your gluteal muscles layer by layer. Although you cannot lose your saddlebags on the outer hip by working them, if you tone the muscle underneath the fat, there is an appearance of spot reduction. This is because the overlying fat is stretched over a greater surface due to your increased muscle tone. Your outer hips appear thinner, although the total amount of fat stays the same.

Place your right hand on the side of your right hip. Raise your right leg out to the right side. The muscle that you feel flexing is your hip abductor. It is part of the upper hip. This is the muscle that firms your saddlebag area. It is also called the gluteus medius.

The *gluteus medius* lies under the gluteus maximus and adds to the roundness of your butt. This muscle connects from the upper pelvis to the upper edge of your thighbone. The gluteus minimus is a smaller muscle that lies underneath the gluteus medius.

These muscles are easy to tone up using isolation exercises. But their most important function is to balance your movement during lunges and squats. These balancing muscles help with other glute-toning activities that you do outside of the gym, such as walking and hiking.

Inner Thighs

If you were asked to demonstrate your muscularity, you would probably flex your upper arm rather than your inner thigh. Flabby inner thighs are common. Fat and muscle are two separate entities and there is no magic formula to change fat into muscle.

You can't change how your muscles attach, your bone structure, or other hereditary factors, but you can certainly change the overall shape and definition of your inner thighs and improve your symmetry. You can sculpt your inner thigh muscles into a work of art.

Your inner thigh muscles are found deep in the inner groin and along the inner thigh. They are noticeably larger than the hamstrings and are almost as big as the quads. Your inner thigh muscles are easy to feel with your own hands. Place the palm of your hand on the inside of your thigh. Press your knees together and you will feel the large tendon become firm as the muscles pull taut. Trace the firm shape of the flexed muscles almost all of the way down to your knee.

The five muscles that make up the inner thighs are collectively called the *hip adductors*, named after the movement they perform, which is bringing the legs toward and across the midline of the body. Individually, these muscles are the *adductors magnus, longus,* and *brevis;* the *gracilis;* and the *pectineus.* The latter two are also hip flexor muscles.

All five muscles attach from the pubis bone and ischial tuberosities (sit bones) and connect to the thighbone. Two of the adductors, the pectineus and the adductor brevis, are quite short and are connected to the back of the upper thighbone. The adductor longus and adductor magnus are longer and larger, and connect at the back of the lower thighbone. The longest adductor, the gracilis, inserts below the knee, on the inner upper shinbone. Together, all five of these muscles pull the thighs together. Several of them also have good leverage to flex the hip, pulling the thigh and torso toward each other.

The inner thigh muscles help you to keep your balance and are used for walking, standing, or climbing. The other actions of the inner thigh muscles are quite complicated. Depending on the position of the leg, they may also help rotate the thighbone internally or externally in the hip socket, or help straighten the hip.

These options provide you with multiple ways to train them to become firm and toned. Read Chapters 4 through 6 to do just that.

Chapter 2

Noodling Bun-damentals

In This Chapter

- Motivation to change
- Do it, and do it right
- No pain is gain
- Work out smart

Turn around and look at yourself in the mirror and decide if you're in shape. Although your thighs and buns may have turned to mush, there *is* a shape underneath the fluff. You may not be in the best shape of your life, but so what? Today is your starting point. Prepare to totally focus on firming those buns and thighs.

Brain Training Is Key

Making the decision to change is a huge first step. Choose your goal: a round, lifted bottom; or just to be able to slide into your jeans. Be specific. For example, set a goal of losing a pants or dress size in two weeks. Quick goals keep you motivated to stick it out. Don't worry about how long it takes. You may also want to set a long-term goal and use the quick goals as points reaching toward that goal.

Plan your battle of the buns. Are you going to work out by yourself, with friends, or both? Can you begin tomorrow? Do you prefer long walks alone or socializing at the gym? Can you stick to one activity, or do you prefer to cross-train?

 Your Personal Trainer

Partner training is great for your motivation. Choose a reliable partner.

You never will know how firm and toned your buns and thighs can be until you begin working out. You may have awesome genetic potential, but you have to give yourself a chance. Motivation must come from inside you. At first, you may exercise because you want to look good for your significant other. But do it for yourself and you will stay with the program.

Before you begin, think about how your buns and thighs will look after you have been on this program for a month. It will feel great to have a lower body you can be proud of. Pull your shoulders back and sit up tall, knowing that your toned thighs are just around the corner. Create a detailed mental picture of your ideal defined legs. It also helps to find a picture of someone you admire that you are built similar to, for help in visualizing the change in your body.

Working In Your Workout

Find a few minutes a day to get your workout in.
Whatever fits your schedule is the best time to work
out. To avoid skipping workouts after work, when
you're tired, or have other obligations, schedule
your training in the AM or at lunchtime. Lunch
break workouts can energize the mid-afternoon
slump. Evening workouts may turn into a social
hour, but that's okay if you combine talking and
training. Decide what type of workout schedule has
worked for you in the past. You might not be a morning person, but nobody can bother you at 6:00 A.M.
Give it a try for a month. You can reset your biologi-
cal clock to an "early to bed, early to rise" mentality.

Consistent eating habits are important, too. Schedule
meals in advance and sit down to all of your meals.
Your disciplined eating improves the more you do
it. The nutrition portion is one of the most important aspects of this program!

You cannot go wrong on this program. Miss a day,
that's okay. Missing a week is required every six
months. For now, the important thing is to find a
few minutes each day.

Any Workout Will Work

Have you started yet? Go by the book on the bun-
and thigh-isolation exercises, but create your own
easy-activity workouts. Any activity that gets you
out of your chair will work. Working out doesn't

have to be work. Take your kids to the playground and do step-ups while they slide. Push them on a swing set and you will feel your buns and thighs flexing as if you were doing lunges in the gym. When you are sedentary, think about ways you could be moving.

Do a little bit of everything to get started. A five-minute walk, five minutes of squats, and a five-minute cool-down stretch is an excellent beginning. "Work out smart, not hard" is a great phrase to remember. Training is not about "the burn" or a couple of days of soreness. But you have to get started. So start today.

Your buns won't firm up after your first workout, but you will feel so much better. Your energy level will increase and you will catch yourself looking over your shoulder in the mirror to measure your progress. Check out the models in this book and copy the form and posture of their movements.

Keeping It Up—and Kicking It Up

Keep your bun- and thigh-toning goals in the back of your mind and you can firm your gorgeous gams all day long. Some great bun-blasting cardio activities include in-line skating, stair climbing, and cycling. The fat around your hips doesn't know whether you are walking or skating. And your muscles will firm up with squats or lunges. Make your workouts a habit. Do not miss any workouts for a month. After a month of easy exercise and eating properly (see

Chapter 8) gauge your progress with a tape measure. Your success deserves a reward. Each month measure your progress and decide how you will spoil yourself (massage, manicure …).

You should give the muscle group you have just trained at least 48 hours rest before training it again. If you are sore from a previous leg workout, take the day off. A day off may be just what you need to attack your leg workout the next day. Every so often give yourself a break just because. A one-day splurge every week or a week off from exercise every six months is necessary. Your body needs an occasional break and so does your mind.

After you have been working out for several months, ask your body how it feels after the workout. Do your thighs prefer to run or skate? Stick to what you and your body like to do. Working out doesn't require discipline. Staying with an exercise program is about having fun.

Follow a consistent routine when you begin your training. Before your squats, adjust the bar on your shoulders, keep your chest out, bring your feet into position, and exhale during each repetition. As you get more advanced you may want to change your training routine up regularly to keep your body "guessing" and to avoid boredom.

Once you begin your workout, don't rush. Impetuous gym-goers strain their knees and backs instead of training their thighs and buns. They struggle so hard to finish reps they are injured for a month.

Join a Gym?

You don't have to join a gym to have fun, but it sure helps. Unless you're extremely disciplined, you're likely to get more accomplished at the gym than at home. Working out at home is tough. You may have distractions such as housework or children that hinder or interrupt your workout.

And the feeling of driving home from the gym with a toned set of buns and thighs can't be beat. Interacting with people who are excited about working out may be just what you need to continue your program.

Leg day at the gym is tough. You are training all of the muscles in your body when you are training your legs. It's great to have someone there to encourage you through your reps. If you do squats, lunges, and dead lifts at a gym, it would be great to have a spotter. Ask for a spot from someone you'd like to befriend, and you may find you have chosen your new workout partner. If you have any questions or need help, ask the gym staff as well.

Get It Right

When someone watches you work out, it gives you extra pep to get a couple of extra reps. Be careful not to lose your form.

Avoiding the Traps

Most people quit exercising because of lack of time, injury, negative emotions, poor social support, or low motivation. This does not have to be you.

Don't start working out too hard or not hard enough. If you can only do three reps of lunges with no weight on the bar, that's a start. Add a rep a week until you can do ten.

There are no absolutes when it comes to training. Target heart rates, strict eating programs, and forced reps are options, not requirements. Re-evaluate your goals so that your exercise strategy is specific to what you really want.

If you don't have much time to work out, break up your program into manageable parts. You can do a great leg workout in just a few minutes using your own body weight. Separate your mini-workouts into manageable segments that fit into your life.

Alternate five minutes of walking in place with five minutes of bun and thigh isolation. Segmenting your workout can actually be more intense because you make the most of those few minutes.

Stay cool no matter what goes wrong with your workout. You won't have a perfect workout each time. Many factors affect your workout. Did you get enough sleep? Have you been feeding your muscles properly? How have your stress levels been? Did you run the day before your leg workout? If something goes wrong during your workout, note it, adjust, and then go on. Keep a training log to help keep track of these factors.

Have a back-up plan for your backside workout. Mentally prepare for unexpected events. Make firming and toning your lower body a priority and you will accomplish your workout goals.

If you strain a leg muscle, see your physician and ask if there is a way to work out around the problem. Show your doctor all of the different exercises in this book so he can help you to continue your progress.

Visualize Your Thighs and Buns

Take a mental snapshot of your ideal buns and streamlined thighs. Now picture the type of training it will take for you to get there. Rehearse doing squats, lunges, dead lifts, good-mornings, and all of your office and home bun and thigh exercises.

Just as you practice a speech before you give it, mentally practicing your workout will help you to perfect your form, and provide you with the motivation to complete your reps.

 Bet You Didn't Know

Just by thinking about doing your leg workout your heart rate may increase by as much as 50 percent.

Use the following exercise to learn to focus on your buns and thighs.

1. Lie down on your back.

2. Press the back of your heels into the floor for three seconds.

3. Feel your thighs, buns, and hamstrings flex.

4. Relax for three seconds.

Continue this cycle of flexing and relaxing for ten repetitions.

This mind-muscle exercise teaches you to be aware of your muscles while you are training them. Then when you are doing your bun- and thigh-isolation exercises, you will notice if you are unnecessarily straining other joints or muscles.

Since you can't see your buns while you are training them, you have to feel the movement and focus on your buns flexing on each repetition. Bodybuilders "see" the range of motion in their mind's eye before they perform the exercise. This mental workout makes leg training easier and more effective.

Place the palms of your hands on your thighs. Imagine yourself doing a set of squats. Feel your thigh muscles flex. Mentally rehearsing squats improves the mind-to-muscle connection.

Imagine performing the perfect squat. Pretend you are standing with your feet shoulder-width apart, your back straight, and your eyes up, and contract your buns. You did it! You actually created a mind-to-muscle connection.

In Other Words _____

Visuo-motor behavior rehearsal (VMBR) is a combination of using relaxation and imagery to improve athletic performance.

Thinking about your leg workout in advance is good. Obsessing about it is counterproductive. Your mind can affect your body in a negative way. Worrying about the effort and intensity required to complete your bun and thigh workout can hurt your progress. Instead, always imagine the benefits of your leg workouts. See yourself as enthusiastic and excited to get started.

Talk to yourself positively during your leg workout. Instead of saying, "I'll never get it," say, "I can get this, and I will." Self-talk such as "My thighs are becoming defined" raises your enthusiasm to keep your mind on your workout and finish your training.

Leg day refers to the day in the week in your workout program where you do lower-body exercises. Leg day is challenging. There is no getting around the fact that your lower-body muscle group is the largest in your body. It takes a lot less effort to train your biceps than your thighs and buns. Your workout requires a lot of physical and mental energy.

That's why you feel so good after training your lower body. You know you have accomplished something special.

Putting It All Together

Keeping a log of your leg workouts can help you to track your progress. Writing down your goals and keeping track of your sets, reps, and how much weight you lifted is proof positive that you are making progress.

Leg workouts require more motivation than other muscle groups. Use your favorite tunes to pump up your efforts. Listen to whatever music gets you in the mood to get those last few reps. Burn your own CDs of motivating rhythms to coincide with the intensity of your workouts. Music can be a huge factor in the quality of your workouts!

Sometimes it's difficult to know how long to rest between sets of squats, lunges, or dead lifts. Discerning between mental and physical fatigue is not easy.

A popular tool to help you more objectively determine if you are ready for your next set is a heart rate monitor (HRM). HRMs are easy to use and are more accurate than taking your pulse from the neck or wrist. When your heart rate drops enough to complete your next set, it will "beep," telling you to get ready.

Use your favorite music, an HRM, VMBR, TV, or whatever it takes to tie those shoes and get moving. And once you start, never stop.

Chapter 3

Backside Benefits

In This Chapter

- Firm buns, thin thighs in 30 days
- Get excited about leg day
- Your legs are your foundation
- Shape and tone your legs and buns

You don't have to set foot inside a gym or buy fancy equipment to train your buns and thighs. All you need is a few minutes a day, three days a week. Combine the buns and thigh exercise program with a smart eating plan and you can drop a dress or pants size in a few weeks.

Firm buns and toned thighs are the foundation for your entire body. Training your buns and thighs works fast. Nothing like visible proof that your program is working!

Tailor your buns and thigh program to meet your needs and goals. Prior to each workout, plan the order of your exercises and the intensity of workout. Get psyched up for each rep.

Form

You can develop shapely legs and lifted buns by putting groceries away, placing dishes in cupboards, putting clothes on closet shelves, lifting pots off the stove, and hoisting children. Every time you bend down your buns and thighs are getting a workout.

Proper form is the secret. Whatever you're doing, maintain perfect form. Breathe normally. Perform all your activities and exercises in a controlled manner and in a comfortable range of motion.

Maintain perfect posture on every exercise.

Keep your stomach in, relax your neck, and keep your back flat (don't arch). Place the palm of your hand just below your navel. Pooch your stomach out as if you were trying to pose for the "before" picture on an infomercial. Then slowly squeeze your lower abs toward your spine using the lower stomach muscles and hold for three seconds. Relax for a few seconds and try it again.

Do this exercise for a few reps. Then, whenever you're performing bun and thigh exercises, remember to flex these muscles before and during all of your reps. This increases your stability so that your legs produce more force. This also helps reduce the risk of injury.

Focus on a specific part of your buns or thigh. For example, to train the side of your hip, lift the leg out to the side. Relax the remainder of your body so a higher percentage of force is exerted behind the specific muscle group you are working.

Never let weight or repetitions dictate form.

If you are training the fronts of your thighs, keep your facial muscles relaxed. Grunt if you want, but the rest of your body should be relaxed. Move smoothly into each repetition with a controlled, yet 100 percent, energized effort.

Go all the way up and down using a full range of motion on each bun and thigh exercise. Ease into your workout. Start with some easy repetitions, then gradually increase the intensity. If you are exerting, exhale during the contraction. Inhale on your short rests between each contraction.

Balance your leg workout for symmetrical develop-ment of your buns and thighs. An unbalanced work-out program can lead to a difference in strength between the fronts and backs of your legs, making you more susceptible to knee injuries. Fortunately, our program includes exercises to train both sides of your legs at the same time.

Speed

Take your time on each repetition. The slower you move, the less momentum, and the more work your muscles are accomplishing. You should be able to stop at any point during your rep.

Take three seconds in both directions.

There are two different parts of each repetition of your bun and thigh workout. One part is called the "positive"—the "up phase" of the repetition. The second part is the "negative," or the "down phase" of the repetition. It is important to come down slowly on the negative phase. Moving slowly on the negative phase will speed your progress to chisel those buns and thighs.

Bet You Didn't Know

> Pause at the bottom of each rep when you do squats, lunges, and dead lifts and you will recruit more muscle fibers from your buns.

Go slower to use more muscle fibers.

Pay attention to the quality of each rep rather than the quantity of reps that you do. If you are too fatigued to finish the negative portion of a rep, then you've completed enough reps of that exercise.

Your bun and thigh muscles respond well when you use good form at a controlled speed. Cheating on your reps leads to injury. Don't compare how much weight you can lift with someone else. Compare you to you.

To add variety, you can manipulate the amount of reps and weight, as well as the type of reps: full range motion along with a half rep.

Resistance

Resistance training tones your buns and thighs.
There is no better way to contour and streamline
your hips than using resistance. You cannot spot-
reduce body fat, but you can tone up your bun and
thigh muscles. Use dumbbells, bands, or your own
body weight to challenge your lower-body muscles.
The squats, lunges, and dead lifts involved in gardening are resistance exercises, too.

Training your buns and thighs with resistance increases your lean muscle mass. The more lean muscle you have, the more calories your body burns.

You may do all of the aerobic exercise that you can
stand, but if you don't weight train you will eventually lose muscle. Muscle is the engine for your
metabolism.

A major factor behind metabolic meltdown is muscle loss. Your metabolism is how many calories your
body uses, even while sleeping, breathing, or reading this book. One of the main factors that determine
your daily calorie burn is the amount of muscle you
have. Muscle tissue is more active than fat tissue,
with each pound burning about 50 calories a day
just to sustain it. By comparison, each pound of
abdominal fat burns only two calories each day.

To shrink a spreading butt, you need resistance
training. The muscle tissue firms up to speed your
sluggish metabolism. Your toned muscle is more
compact than fat.

After age 25 you begin to lose about a half pound of muscle each year. If you don't start toning, you will lose 5 pounds of muscle and replace it with about 15 pounds of fat every decade. No wonder your friends who say they eat the same now as they did in high school are 30 pounds overweight!

You won't get muscle-bound from resistance training. Women are concerned that they will develop huge muscles. Since women don't have high levels of testosterone, they won't get big and bulky. Swimsuit models lift weights, and so did Marilyn Monroe to keep her curvaceous figure.

The key to strength and muscle development is progressive resistance, which is also called the "overload principle." Overloading involves applying a greater-than-normal stress to your bun and thigh muscles. The overload may be in the form of increased weight, reps, sets, or less rest between sets. If an exercise doesn't challenge your muscles with an overload, there is little benefit.

Three important overload factors in your bun and thigh workouts that will dictate your progress are the intensity of the stress put on the muscle, the duration of the training period, and the frequency of the workouts.

If your bun and thigh muscles are feeling stronger and more toned, and you are not gaining additional body fat, you are doing everything right.

In Other Words

Basal metabolic rate (BMR) is the number of calories your body burns at rest. About 25 percent of your BMR is based on how much muscle you have.

Resistance is not necessary for most exercises.

At first, your body weight is enough resistance. Soon your leg muscles will adapt by getting stronger. You should add resistance using bands, free weights, or machine weights. Your eventual goal will be to do 10 reps with about 75 percent of the maximum resistance you can handle for one rep.

Your body weight is enough resistance.

When you begin to use resistance, start with very light weight. When you can perform 10 repetitions with perfect form you can add weight. Increase the resistance no more than 5 percent in a single workout.

Sets

At first, perform one set of each exercise. In addition to being time efficient, single-set training is almost as effective as multiple-set training.

Make sure you don't duplicate movements. For example, it makes no sense to do a set of squats with no resistance, and then another set of squats with resistance bands. Both of these exercises are exactly the same movement and work the same specific muscles. Instead, do a set of squats for your buns and thighs and then a set of lunges that target the balancing muscles on the sides of the hips (saddlebags).

Perform one to three sets per body part.

After you train for a few months, your buns and thigh muscles will get stronger and can handle more than one set of a particular exercise. Add another set for each exercise that you do. When that becomes easy, and after another month of training, work your way up to three sets of each exercise. Three sets is the maximum number of sets you are required to do. Doing more than three sets provides diminishing returns and, worse than that, you might be overtraining.

If you're doing a squat and you start wobbling, you're finished with the exercise. If you break your form during any rep of any set of any exercise, stop the exercise immediately. Losing your form means you can't finish a rep without changing your body position.

Get It Right

Everybody is different concerning how far they can safely descend for squats, lunges, and dead lifts. It depends on limb and torso length and flexibility.

Perform sets consecutively or in a circuit.

When you are ready for a challenge, do a bun and thigh circuit, performing one set of each exercise without rest. This burns more calories than straight sets.

Circuit training also forces your cardiovascular system to work overtime. Without resting between sets, you increase the amount of time you spend toning those legs compared with the amount of time you spend resting. This increases the metabolic demand of the workout while maintaining your strength and tone. You may need a little more recovery/rest time in between super-sets or circuit training intervals because they are more difficult than performing straight sets.

Pulsing through your squats is another way to add intensity. The principle behind pulsing is that instead of doing full-range-of-motion squats, you just stay at your mid-range and do half-squats. Do 3 sets of 10 repetitions, resting 1 minute between each set. Follow that up with a regular set of 10 full-range-of-motion squats. Pulsing preps your body for using more resistance because it allows you to overload the part of your leg muscles that are strongest, without being limited by the part of the movement where you're weakest.

Choose a bun or thigh exercise that you have difficulty doing a single rep of. Perform 10 sets of one repetition, resting 30 seconds between each set. This is a fabulous workout because you end up performing 10 repetitions of an exercise you normally can only do 1 or 2 reps of. This program requires you to recruit more total muscle fibers than usual.

Take your current set and rep scheme and reverse it. Since you normally do 3 sets of 10 reps, try squatting 10 sets of 3 reps. Since you're stopping at 3 reps instead of 10, rest 10 seconds or less between sets. Reversing your sets and reps allows you to do the same number of total repetitions, but increases the average amount of force your muscles apply during the exercise.

Cut your workout in half. Believe it or not, you may be overtraining your legs. By reducing the demand on them, you'll allow them to recover. Another option would be to take a week off. When you come back stronger after this leg break, you'll know you were overtraining.

Giant sets consist of performing three different exercises for your legs consecutively. For example, do a set of squats followed by lunges and dead lifts with minimal rest in between.

A superset is performing 2 different exercises for opposing muscle groups consecutively. Do a set of 10 reps for your thighs followed immediately by a set of 10 reps for your hamstrings. Or you could do a set of step-ups on a bench followed by a set of good-mornings.

Reps

If you increase the number of reps you can do with good form, you have increased your strength and most likely the muscle tone in your buns and thighs as well. But doing hundreds of squats in a single workout doesn't adequately challenge your muscles.

First of all, you are probably not performing perfect squats, and secondly, if you can do hundreds of squats with perfect form, you're overdue for adding resistance.

Doing hundreds of repetitions is kind of like chewing gum. You don't get a trimmed, toned jaw if you chew a lot of gum.

Do at least 10 repetitions of each exercise.

The overload principle increases the strength of your buns and thighs, but it's also essential for boosting your metabolism and maximizing your rate of fat loss.

When you train your legs, you damage your muscle fibers. After your workout, your body repairs those fibers, a process that requires calories.

Added resistance to your leg training requires you to use more muscle fibers. You'll increase the number of fibers that are damaged and use more calories after you've finished your workout to repair them.

Do fewer reps for strength.

Add enough weight to challenge your buns and
thighs, but not enough to compromise your form.

Do more reps for endurance.

Complete 10 to 12 repetitions with 75 percent of
your maximum resistance if your goal is muscular
endurance. Ten reps is a good compromise of both
absolute strength and muscular endurance.

Rest

Training your legs two days a week is more than
enough. Figure out which days will work best in your
busy schedule. Spread your days out to get enough
rest in between your workouts. Tuesday and Friday
works great. Stick with the days that allow you the
best chance of being consistent. These should be
designated as your official bun and thigh–toning days.

Your Personal Trainer

If you do a lot of running or cycling,
you may only need to train your legs
once a week. If you're stronger when
you cut out one of your leg-workout days,
once is enough.

Rest no longer than a minute between sets.

During your rest period, blood delivers oxygen and energy to your legs and carries away waste products. When you first begin a leg-training program, the best ratio of rest to work is three parts rest to one part leg training. This is about a two-minute cycle with leg work being done in the first 30 seconds and rest for the remaining minute and a half.

Rest longer for heavy sets and shorter for light sets.

Keep track of how much time you rest between sets during your bun and thigh workout. As your conditioning improves, perform the same total number of sets and reps, but lessen your rest periods to a maximum of 60 seconds. This requires your muscles to recover faster between sets and increases your results.

The heavier the set, the more rest you need. One way to minimize the rest time between sets is to superset thigh and hamstring exercises. Do a set of one-legged squats for the fronts of your legs followed immediately by a set of butt blasters for your hamstrings and buns. While the front of your leg is working, the back is resting and vice versa.

Take at least two days rest between workouts.

Your leg muscles should be given 48 to 72 hours of rest before attacking them again. Your muscles firm up between training days. However, too much rest between workouts can hurt your progress. In as little as 96 hours, the benefits of all of your hard leg work can begin to disappear.

Chapter 4

Home-Work

In This Chapter

- Home-made buns and thighs
- Home foundation training
- Lift your buns
- Super toning for visible results

Your buns and thighs are the foundation of your body. And there's no better place to build a foundation than in your living room. Bun and thigh training at home is an adventure in creative exercise. Perform traditional squats and lunges, but you can also firm your buns and thighs while climbing stairs and doing chores. Tone your buns and thighs throughout the day or designate a specific time for your training. If you choose the latter, let the answering machine take your calls, have water available, lock the doors, and begin.

On all home bun and thigh exercises, keep your back straight and stomach in. Imagine a piece of dental floss tied around your waist while performing every exercise. Use your lower abs to flex your navel in toward your spine. Exhale on the exertion of each rep. Keep your neck relaxed and maintain your concentration throughout each repetition.

Lift a Pencil Off the Floor

Lifting a pencil off the floor doesn't seem like much of an exercise, but it is the perfect movement to train your buns and thighs. In fact, consider *any* lifting movement as a buns and thigh toner.

The hard part about doing this exercise is to maintain perfect form when it's a lot easier to cheat by bending from your waist. Although the pencil is not very heavy, use perfect form through the movement. When most people pick up a pencil from the floor, they bend and twist their spine—not very healthy for your back. Keep your head up, chest out, and stomach in. Bend your knees and lead with your hips.

In Other Words

Your gluteus maximus (glutes) refers to your buns while your quadriceps (quads) are the four large muscles on the front of your thigh.

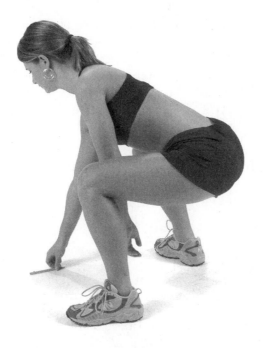

1. Move in close to the pencil and spread your feet at least shoulder-width apart.

2. Squat as if into a chair and pick up the pencil.

Free Squat

The Free Squat is the single best exercise to isolate your buns, thighs, hamstrings, and outer and inner thighs. Squat as if you were sitting back into a chair. Keep your upper body lifted with your shoulders back and head up. Always lead with your hips. There is no need to squat past a position where your thighs are parallel to the floor. Be sure that your knees do not travel over your toes and keep your knees in line with your toes. Don't worry how far you descend. That will depend on your limb and torso length and your flexibility. If you begin to lean forward, or your knees draw inward, return to your starting position.

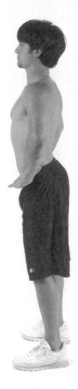

1. Place your hands on your hips and spread your feet shoulder-width apart. Keep your chest out and eyes looking over the horizon.

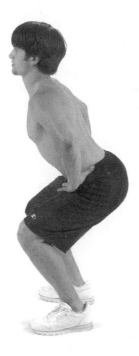

2. Press through your heels and sit back as if into a chair until your thighs are parallel to the floor. If your knees begin to travel over your toes or you lose your form, stop immediately and slowly move back into your original position.

Lunge

The Lunge firms your thighs, buns, hamstrings, and inner and outer thighs. The Lunge is an athletic move that requires you to use balancing muscles. Pull your shoulders back and toward each other. Stay perfectly aligned so the exercise targets your legs and buns instead of your lower back. Keep your chest and head up. Resist the temptation to look down at your feet. Imagine an apple tucked between your chin and your chest.

Focus on your front leg as the workhorse for this exercise. Your back leg is there for balance. Don't go down too far if you have any problems with your knees or ankles. Maintain a 90 degree angle with your ankle, knee, and hip. Be sure your knees do not travel beyond your toes. At first, you may just bend down to a 45 degree angle with your knees. As you get stronger, you may descend to a position of 90 degrees.

Your Personal Trainer

Do squats and lunges whenever you can because they are the best exercises to firm all of your bun and thigh muscles, including your inner and outer thighs.

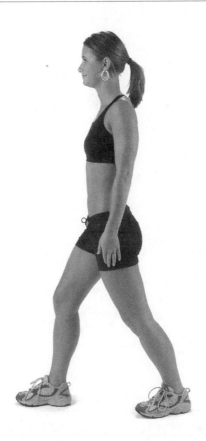

1. Step forward with your right foot as if you were straddling a railroad track. Keep your chest out and eyes forward.

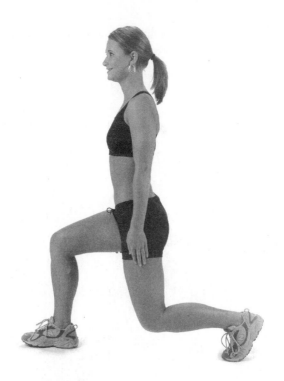

2. Press through the heel of your front foot. Bend both knees to a 90 degree angle. Be sure your knees do not travel beyond your toes. Switch legs and repeat.

Chores

Chores such as loading the dishwasher tone your thighs, buns, hamstrings, and inner and outer thighs if you bend down with perfect form. Simulate squats and lunges on every lifting or lowering movement.

You can get a great workout in the kitchen. Keep your center of gravity over your hips.

Whether you are putting away dishes or lifting a watermelon from the bottom of the refrigerator, move slowly and purposefully, as if you were in slow motion. Concentrate on the muscles that are working. Be careful not to reach or rush through the movements. Treat these movements with the same care that you would any other exercise.

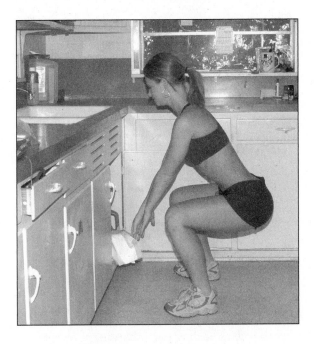

1. Get as close as possible to the dishwasher. Bend from your hips, knees, and ankles.

2. Instead of reaching, step into your lift.

Climbing Stairs

Climbing stairs tones your thighs, buns, hamstrings, and inner and outer thighs. If you have stairs in your home, you don't need a stair-climbing machine. Focus on toning your thighs by staying on the balls of your feet. To firm your buns, press through your heels on each step. Use the handrails for balance only. Do not pull on the handrails.

For advanced stepping, walk upstairs backward. Use the handrail for balance until you master this technique. Keep your form perfect, just as you would for any other exercise. Move in slow motion. As a change of pace you may side-step up and down the stairs. Train the same muscles at different angles.

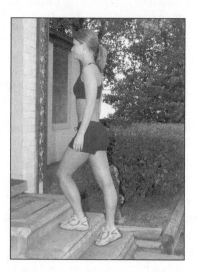

1. Use the handrail for balance, step through your heel, and keep your head and chest up.

Get It Right _____

Train your thighs and hamstrings equally to prevent a muscle imbalance which could cause a knee injury.

Back Wall Press

The Back Wall Press firms your buns and hamstrings. (This was a punishment exercise in elementary school!) While your hips are against the wall you have the choice to target-tone your thighs or your hamstrings. For thigh work, center your weight on the balls of your feet. To burn your buns, shift your weight to your heels.

To train both your thighs and buns, shift your weight back and forth. Keep your eyes forward, shoulders down, and your upper body relaxed. Your back should retain its natural curve. If your knees bother you on this exercise, bend your knees at 45 degrees instead of 90 degrees.

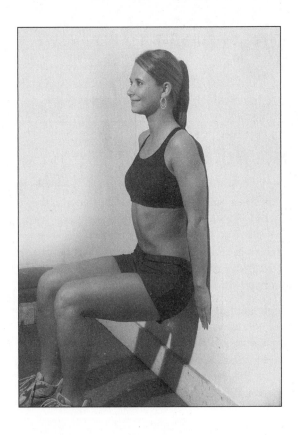

1. Stand with your back against a wall and slowly lower your hips until your knees are bent at 90 degrees.

2. Press through your heels in order to target your buns.

Lying on Your Back Buns Blaster

The Lying on Your Back Buns Blaster targets your buns and hamstrings. Do not arch your back or lift your hips too high. This is a great exercise to do when you don't want people to know you're working out; it's a very subtle movement.

On each rep, draw your navel into your spine and hold the contraction throughout the duration of the exercise. This exercise may be accomplished with both legs or one leg at a time. You can do this while watching television or reading in bed.

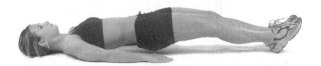

1. Lie on your back with your legs together and your knees slightly bent.

2. Press your heels into the floor and hold for three seconds.

 In Other Words

Resistance training is the best tool to reshape your buns and thighs. Cardio is second best.

Lying on Your Stomach Buns Blaster

Lying on Your Stomach Buns Blaster trains your buns and hamstrings. Begin this exercise by drawing your navel into your spine. Flex your buns as you begin to lift your legs off of the floor. Lift them no higher than an inch off of the floor. Be careful not to hold your breath on this exercise. Instead, exhale through pursed lips throughout each rep.

If this exercise feels too difficult, do one leg at a time and alternate legs. After you have mastered this exercise and are ready for a challenge, add some weight to your ankles.

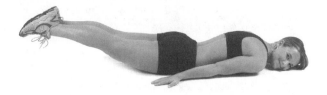

1. Lie on your stomach with your arms to your sides. Turn your head to one side.

2. Lift your legs and be sure you are hinging from your hip. Hold for three seconds.

Side Wall Press

The Side Wall Press firms the outside of your hips (saddlebags). If this muscle doesn't get enough stimulation it loses its tone. A toned hip muscle adds shape to your bottom. As you get stronger, you may press harder into the wall. Pressing harder is like adding weight on a weight machine. At first, hold on to the wall with your hand for balance.

Begin each exercise by drawing your navel into your spine. Flex the side of your hip to begin the movement. Exhale through the duration of each rep.

After you have mastered the exercise, allow your supporting leg to provide stability and let go with your hand. When you can do this exercise without holding on, you are training the outside of the hips of both legs simultaneously. Pay attention to your posture and keep your upper body relaxed.

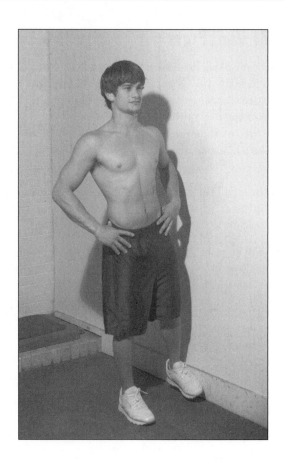

1. Stand straight, with your right foot three inches away from a wall. Your right side is facing the wall.

2. Press the edge of your right foot into the wall and hold for three seconds. Switch legs and repeat.

Back Heel Press

The Back Heel Press firms your buns and hamstrings. Begin each exercise by drawing your navel into your spine. Similar to the side wall press, gradually increase how hard you press against the wall. Keep your back straight and exhale through the duration of each rep.

For this exercise, do not hold on to the wall for balance. Allow your supporting leg to stabilize your movement. This gives your supporting leg a workout, too. Maintain perfect posture and focus on firming your buns.

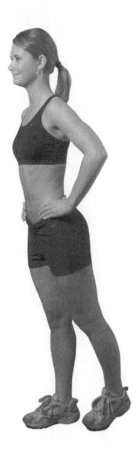

1. Stand three inches in front of a wall and extend your right leg back until the back edge of your heel makes contact.

2. Press and hold for three seconds. Switch legs and repeat.

5

Office Slim-Down

In This Chapter

- Working out while you work
- Small movements, big results
- Toning and firming under the desk
- Shrink those thighs

Secretary spread is sweeping the nation, and not just for women. Sitting all day long is the worst thing you can do if you want to have great buns and thighs. Wouldn't it be great if you could firm your buns and thighs in your office chair while you're reading or typing?

Well, you can, and it's easy! You can even do these simple exercises while on the phone or during a live interview. All of the movements are subtle, but the toning and shaping effects are amazing.

Maintain perfect posture on every exercise. Be sure to breathe normally while you flex your target muscle. Hold each squeeze for 3 seconds. Perform 10 reps of each exercise. Keep your upper body relaxed. At first, while you're in the learning stage, concentrate fully on your form. After a few months you will be able to firm and tone while you multitask on your computer or conduct an interview.

Heel Press

The Heel Press firms your thighs, buns, and hamstrings. There's no learning curve on this great start-up exercise. Your office mates will have no idea you're toning your lower body. At first, press lightly into the floor. As you get stronger, challenge yourself to press harder. Breathe normally or exhale into each rep. Flex your lower abs into your spine to get even better results. Eventually you will feel as if you might be able to rise up out of the chair without using your armrests.

Keep your back straight and your head up. Wear flat shoes or kick them off. High heels won't work very well for this exercise. To spice things up, isolate each leg by performing alternating heel presses.

In Other Words

The sides of your hips (saddlebags) known as your gluteus medius balance your movement when you walk or do lunges and squats.

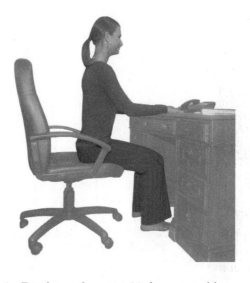

1. Bend your knees at 90 degrees and keep your feet flat on the floor.

2. Press your heels into the floor.

Outer Thigh Press

The Outer Thigh Press firms the sides of your hips (saddlebags) and buns. It's amazing how much you can firm and tone these muscles in the privacy of your office. You can also do this exercise while you're in a meeting or on the phone. After you practice for a couple of weeks, your effort will be undetectable to others.

You can breathe normally or exhale into each rep. Flex your lower abs into your spine to get even better results. As you get stronger and are looking for a further challenge, press harder. Do not hunch over. Use your armrests to brace your effort if necessary. As a change of pace, alternate legs.

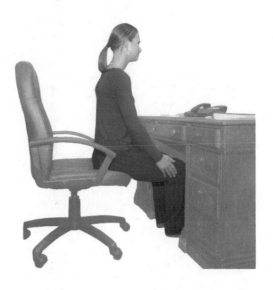

1. Sit at the front of your chair with your knees bent at 90 degrees and your feet together.

2. Place your hands on the outside of your knees and press the outside of your knees against your hands.

Figure-4 Press

The Figure-4 Press tones your outer thighs and buns. If someone saw you in this position, it would just look like you were relaxing or in deep thought. Little do they know you're spot-toning your hips and saddlebags!

Be careful not to press too hard. Breathe normally or exhale into each rep. Flex your lower abs into your spine to get even better results. At first, use your arms to brace yourself if necessary. Adjust your ankle on your thigh to change the angle of the exercise. This recruits muscles at different angles to further your progress. At first, alternate legs after each rep. After a month of doing the exercise at least twice a week, perform all 10 reps on one side, then all 10 reps on the other side. Take as much rest as you need between reps.

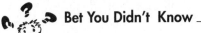 **Bet You Didn't Know**

Fixing flabby inner thighs is as much a function of a proper diet as firming the muscle underneath the fat with toning exercises.

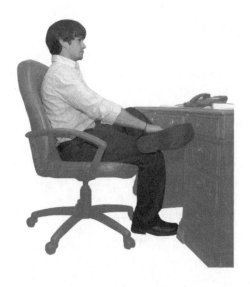

1. Sit in a Figure-4 position with your right ankle resting on your left knee.

2. Press your ankle into your thigh. Repeat with your other leg.

Cross Ankle

The Cross Ankle firms your outer thighs and buns. This is another great exercise that is imperceptible to others. Don't squeeze too tight at first. Breathe normally or exhale into each rep. Flex your lower abs into your spine to get even better results.

As you become stronger, squeeze harder. Do not lean forward or back on this exercise. At first, alternate legs after each rep. After a month of doing this exercise at least twice a week, perform all 10 reps on one side, then all 10 reps on the other side. Take as much rest as you need between reps.

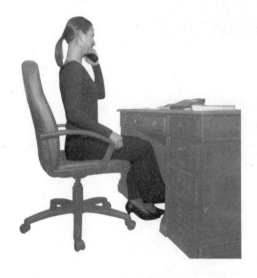

1. Cross your right ankle over your left ankle with your knees together.

2. Press the outside edges of your feet together.

3. Cross your left ankle over your right ankle and repeat.

T-Press

The T-Press is a firming exercise for your inner thighs and hamstrings. In this exercise, both legs are working, so be sure to maintain perfect form and posture. Since both feet are resisting each other, there is a toning effect for both legs.

At first, alternate legs between reps. After a month of doing this exercise at least twice a week, perform all 10 reps on one side, then all 10 reps on the other side. Take as much rest as you need between reps. Breathe normally or exhale into each rep. Flex your lower abs into your spine to get even better results.

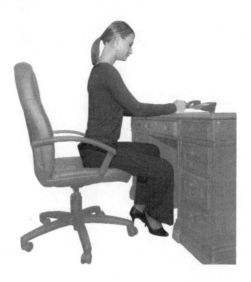

1. Sit with your left foot pointed straight ahead and your left knee bent at 90 degrees.

2. Place the back heel of your right foot into the inside middle of your left foot. Your right foot should be pointed to the right and your right knee is slightly bent.

3. Press the back of your right heel into the middle of your left foot.

4. Switch legs and repeat.

Your Personal Trainer

When performing your bun and thigh exercises, keep equal pressure on both legs to maintain proper symmetry and a shapely, balanced look.

V-Press

The V-Press shapes your buns and inner thighs. At first, simply concentrate on pressing your heels together with your toes pointed outward. As you become more advanced, you may benefit your pelvic floor muscles while you perform this exercise by doing a Kegal. A Kegal is when you squeeze the muscles that you would use to stop urinating. To receive even greater benefit on this exercise, squeeze your bun cheeks together.

Breathe normally or exhale into each rep. Maintain perfect posture.

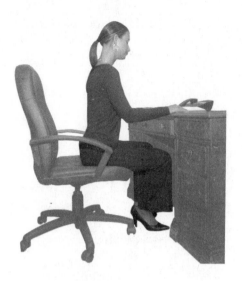

1. Sit with your heels together and your toes pointed slightly outward.

2. Press the inside of your heels together.

3. At the same time, press your heels into the floor.

Bow-Legged

The Bow-Legged firms your inner thighs and buns. Do not slouch on this exercise. Be careful not to press too hard at first. Your inner thigh muscles are probably not used to this type of a workout. You may breathe normally or exhale into each rep.

Flex your lower abs into your spine to get even better results. Press lightly at first, and then as you get stronger you may press harder. Apply equal pressure with both legs.

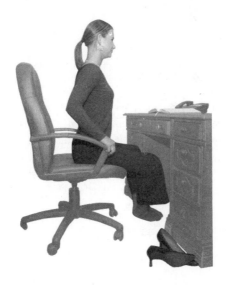

1. Sit with the soles of your feet together and your knees bowed out.

2. Press the soles of your feet together.

Get It Right

Between sets of leg exercises stand up and move around occasionally to get the kinks out and to speed the circulation in your lower body.

Inner Knee Press

The Inner Knee Press tones your inner thighs. No one will know that you are performing this exercise. Press your knees together until you feel tension. Breathe normally or exhale into each rep. Flex your lower abs into your spine to get even better results. As you get stronger, squeeze harder. Use your armrests for balance if necessary.

Maintain perfect posture through the duration of this exercise.

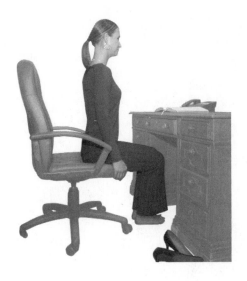

1. Sit with your feet and knees together.

2. Press your knees together.

Chapter 6

Gym Tune-Up

In This Chapter

- Transform and tone your thighs
- Look great fast, get your butt back
- Easy to follow bun and thigh toners
- Slenderizing stretches

Don't be afraid of the gym. If you're concerned that you're the only one with sagging buns or flabby thighs, look around. Most people in the gym are just like you, trying to get to that next level: toned and tight. The most important thing is walking through the doors to make the commitment for your training program. Intimidation should not be a factor—most people are too absorbed in themselves and their own workout to pay attention to you!

Motivated gym-goers can inspire you when you would rather sit on the couch. Gyms are like social clubs—a place to meet new people—and many offer personal training and aerobics classes. If your gym is part of a chain, you can use their facilities in different cities. Gym machines have built-in safety features so that when you can no longer press a weight, you just set it down. Machines remove balance as a factor and ensure correct movements to isolate your buns and thighs. Changing the resistance on a machine is as easy as changing the pin.

Always maintain perfect posture. Keep your back straight, stomach in, chest out, and eyes forward. You will notice as many people doing exercises incorrectly as those training with proper form. It's especially important to maintain proper form when you're training your legs because of the potential for knee or back strain. Never sacrifice form for the amount of weight that you are lifting, and take your time between sets.

During each exercise, bring your navel toward your spine by flexing your lower-abdominal muscles. Move slowly on each repetition—three seconds up, three seconds down. Breathe normally unless you prefer to exhale during the exertion phase. If your legs are still sore from a previous workout, take the day off or do some easy activity. If you feel a twinge of pain on any exercise, stop immediately and seek the advice of your physician.

 In Other Words

Your thighs are named quadriceps because they are made up of four muscles in the fronts of your legs.

Roman Chair Hip Extension

The Roman Chair Hip Extension is a great exercise for your buns. You may perform this exercise with a partner or on a leg-curl or hip-extension machine. Be sure you are hinging at the hip and not the waist. Don't move your upper body too far in either direction. Only go down a few inches below parallel and then come back up a few inches past the parallel position. Place your arms across your chest.

If this exercise is too challenging, use your arms to help press your body into the up position. Take your time—three seconds up and three seconds down works great. If that's too difficult, one second up and one second down is fine as long as your range of motion is only an inch or so.

If placing your arms across your chest is not challenging enough, interlock your fingers behind your head. Breathe normally throughout the entire range of motion of this exercise. If you have back problems, choose a different exercise. You can add a weight across your chest to increase the intensity of the exercise.

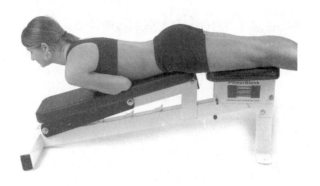

1. Place the backs of your ankles underneath the foot pad and your hips should straddle the pad in front.

2. Place your arms across your chest and allow gravity to let your body descend.

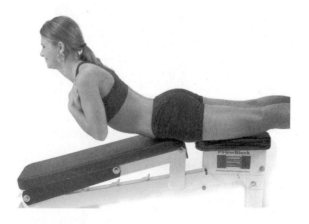

3. Flex your buns and raise your upper body back up to a parallel position.

Your Personal Trainer

Train both your fast- and slow-twitch thigh and bun muscles in the same week by doing 10 to 12 reps one workout with lighter weight, and doing 6 to 8 reps on your next workout with heavier weight.

Stiff-Legged Dead Lifts

Stiff-Legged Dead Lifts are one of the best exercises you can do to firm your buns and hamstrings. Use very light weight or no weight at all when beginning this routine. Be sure your back doesn't round out. Press through your heels to target your buns and hamstrings. Consciously focus on flexing your buns and hamstrings.

You must keep your back straight, chest out, stomach in, and shoulders back when you do this exercise. Visualize a steel rod that goes up your back to help keep proper form on this exercise. Breathe normally or, if you prefer, you may exhale during the up phase of this lift. If you're currently suffering from back pain, do a different exercise instead. Try the lying on your stomach buns blaster exercise from Chapter 4. This exercise firms your buns and strengthens your back. Be sure to get your doctor's approval before you try it.

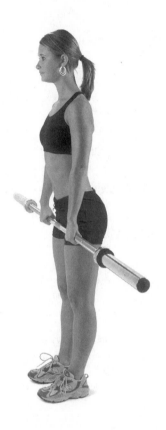

1. Stand with your feet a little less than shoulder-width apart, knees slightly bent, and grab the weights with an overhand grip.

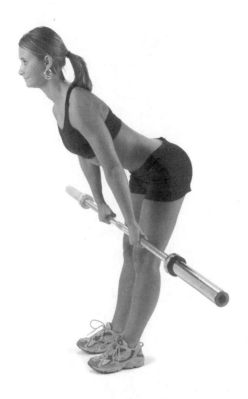

2. Slowly descend until you feel a light stretch in your hamstrings and buns. Keep the weights as close to your legs as possible.

3. Flex your buns and hamstrings and move back to your original position.

Good-Mornings

Good-Mornings train your buns and hamstrings. At first, use very light weight or no weight at all. As you progress, gradually increase weight, but not at the expense of perfect form. You must keep your back straight, head up, and shoulders back when you perform this exercise. Keep your head level and don't raise it up as you lean forward; this will reduce strain during the exercise. Press through your heels and keep both knees slightly bent. Consciously focus on flexing your buns and hamstrings. If you're currently suffering from back pain, do a different exercise, such as the hip extension explained next.

Bet You Didn't Know

Training your legs with weights is a full-body exercise because many muscles in your upper body are used to stabilize your movement.

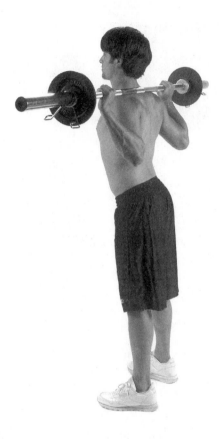

1. Stand with your feet a little less than shoulder-width apart, knees slightly bent, and hold the weight on the back of your shoulders.

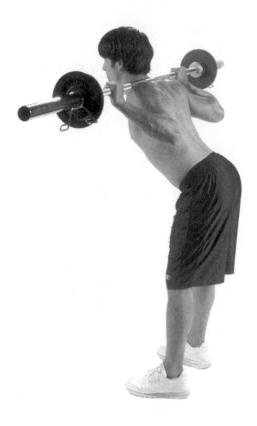

2. Flex your buns and hamstrings as you hinge from the hip and lean forward a few inches.

3. Move back to your original position.

Hip Extension

The Hip Extension tones your buns and hamstrings. Use very light weight to begin with. When you can perform 10 reps with perfect form, add weight. Move 3 seconds up and 3 seconds down. If that is too difficult, 1 second up and 1 second down is fine.

At first, alternate legs. As you become stronger, you may perform all of your sets with one leg before switching to the other leg. Eventually you may perform this exercise lifting both legs simultaneously. Breathe normally or if you prefer, exhale on the up phase. Be careful not to lift your legs more than an inch or two.

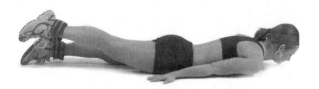

1. Lie on your stomach and place your arms by your sides. Attach the weights to the backs of your ankles. Lift your right leg three inches off of the floor, hinging from the hip. Switch legs and repeat.

One-Legged Quarter-Squat with Dumbbells

The One-Legged Quarter-Squat with Dumbbells firms up your thighs, buns, hamstrings, and inner/outer thighs. You're working the legs in front when you perform this exercise. Be sure not to bend farther than a 90 degree angle with your front knee. Press through your heel to target the back of your leg and buns. Breathe normally or exhale on the up phase if you prefer. Begin with very light weight. It is advisable to have a wall next to you for balance.

Get It Right

Keeping your back straight really means maintaining a natural curve in your lower back. This keeps your spinal disks healthy and prevents injury.

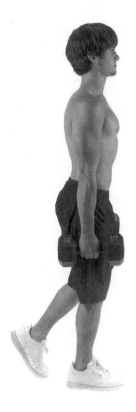

1. Begin in a lunge position with your right
   foot forward and a dumbbell in each hand.

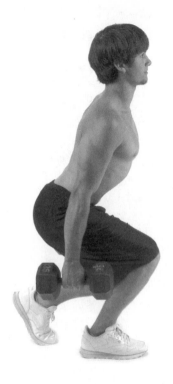

2. Extend your right leg pushing from your heel. Your left leg is there for the purpose of balance only.

3. Switch legs and repeat.

Step-Ups with a Bench

Step-Ups with a Bench work your thighs, buns, hamstrings, and inner/outer thighs. Choose a low bench and maintain your balance throughout the exercise. Your bench should be low enough that you do not shift your body weight using momentum.

Breathe normally or if you prefer, exhale during the up phase. You should be able to hold your position at any point during your repetition. Maintain perfect posture and resist the urge to lean too far forward as you step up. Press through your heels to train the backs of your leg or press through the balls of your feet to focus on your thighs.

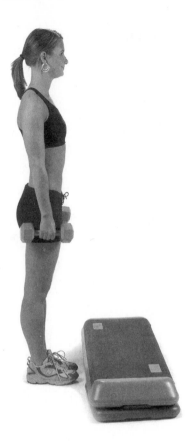

1. Stand in front of a low bench with a dumb-bell in each hand.

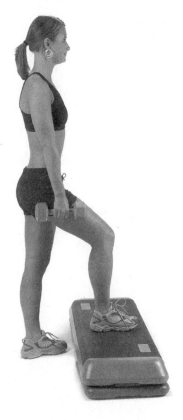

2. Step onto the bench with your right foot and let your left foot swing naturally so that you are standing on the bench with both feet. Step down with your right foot and then step down with your left foot.

3. Step onto the bench with your left foot and let your right foot swing naturally so that you are standing on the bench with both feet. Step down with your left foot and then step down with your right foot.

Single-Legged Squat with a Bench

The Single-Legged Squat with a Bench works your thighs, buns, hamstrings, and inner and outer thighs. It requires strength, flexibility, and balance—that's why this is such a great exercise!

Try this exercise without weight. At first, alternate legs. When you feel strong enough, try 10 repetitions with one leg and then switch to the other. When you can successfully perform 10 repetitions with perfect form with either leg, hold a light dumbbell in each hand. Move as slowly as you can for the duration of this exercise.

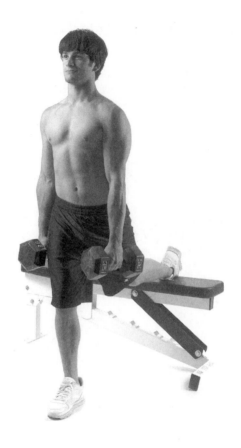

1. Stand with your left foot on a low bench and
   your right foot on the floor. Hold a set of
   dumbbells in each hand.

2. Press your left heel into the bench to raise
   your body up until your right foot taps the
   bench. Don't lock your knee out when you
   rise from the squat.

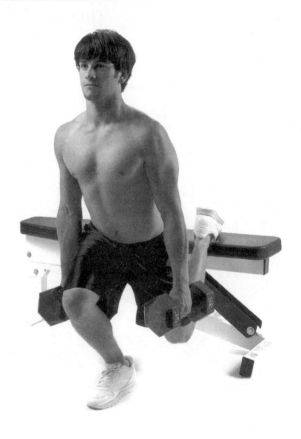

3. Lower yourself slowly to the floor and complete ten repetitions.

4. Switch legs and repeat.

7

Burn It Up

In This Chapter

- Melt fat from your hips and thighs
- Shed fat in all the right places
- Best bun burners
- Stretch and tone buns and thighs
- Jaw-dropping buns can be yours

Losing the fat that surrounds your buns and thighs is easier than you may think. It's not about working in your "target heart rate range." You are burning fat while you read this book.

The way to melt fat is to move. Did you know that you could burn up to 600 calories a day just by fidgeting? In this chapter you will learn to accelerate fat loss doing your favorite activities.

Your Favorite Sitcom Is Your Workout

Work out while you watch your favorite TV show. In an hour-long program there are about 15 minutes of commercials. Simply get off of the couch during each commercial and move.

A minute or two of squats and lunges will have you huffing and puffing. Maintain perfect form and alternate 10 reps of squats and 10 reps of lunges with each leg. Move through that cycle until the commercial is over. You will be glad there is a long break until your next set.

You may also dance, jump rope, do jumping jacks, walk, march, or run in place. The fat surrounding your hips doesn't know the difference between activities.

Bet You Didn't Know

> You may do easy activity and cardio every day. But weight training should be limited to twice a week per muscle group.

The harder you work, the sooner your buns and thighs will take shape. But it doesn't happen in one workout. If you do 100 squats during a 2-minute commercial break, you won't be able to get off the couch for the next commercial.

March in place between squats to reinvigorate your legs.

Indoor Training

Whether you use a treadmill, stair climber, elliptical machine, ski machine, or a stationary bike, choose the activity that you love. All of these devices are useful for firming and sculpting your thighs and buns.

A treadmill is the most popular piece of home fitness equipment, but if you work out on a ski machine, you use more muscle groups and may potentially burn more calories.

Elliptical machines are so popular in gyms that waiting lines are common. A nice feature of elliptical training is that you can move the pedals forward or backward. You can also change the stride length to accommodate for your height on certain machines.

Cross-training keeps you fresh. Pedal one day, climb the next. Walk, jog, or run on a treadmill. Change the pace depending on how you feel. Go fast on a good day. If you don't feel like working out, warm up and then enjoy an easy stroll. Variety is the key to prevent boredom during your workouts!

If walking on a treadmill makes you feel like a gerbil, and pedaling on a stationary bike gets you nowhere, do household chores. Vacuuming, sweeping, mopping, or washing windows burns fat and tones those thighs and buns. Your legs are your foundation for every movement you make. Next time you're loading the dishwasher, notice that the muscles in your legs are flexed. You are firming and toning without knowing it!

Get It Right

Be careful not to develop an overuse injury. One of the greatest predictors of developing another injury is if you are suffering from a current injury.

Outdoor Training

Cavemen spent all day hunting and gathering. Most of us don't even spend 5 minutes a day outdoors. When you get home from work tomorrow, rather then stepping through your front door, go for a 10-minute walk—5 minutes out, 5 minutes back. Do that everyday. Each week add 2 minutes until you are walking for 45 minutes. This is one of the best ways to whittle away the fat that surrounds your buns and thighs.

Your Personal Trainer

Breathe from your belly (diaphragm). You can get more air into your lungs if you belly-breathe.

Once you start adding general activity into your routine, you'll find that a little goes a long way. A couple of brisk 10-minute walks a day are enough for you to lose a couple of inches around your waist in a few months, and that's without changing your diet.

If you're overweight and have not worked out since high school, and you have the good fortune to belong to a gym, begin on a recumbent bicycle. The recumbent bike allows you to lean back to support your body weight. This requires you to work only against the resistance of the bike without having to support your body weight.

Breathing is also easier for some people on a recumbent. Since your legs are up higher than a normal stationary bike, and they are pedaling horizontally, there is less stress to your cardiovascular system. Recumbent bikes are also great for people who've had previous knee injuries.

After you have mastered the recumbent bicycle, move to upright cycling. Upright cycling is more demanding, but it still supports your body weight.

Treadmill walking at an easy pace without an incline is your next step. After you have mastered treadmill walking at an easy pace, increase the grade to one percent. Walking at a one percent grade is challenging. But your body will adapt. When it does, increase your pace.

Next is the stair-stepping machine. (These machines are also called stepmills.) This vertical movement pattern burns more calories and is very challenging, so be patient with your progress.

Stair stepping is one stage below stair climbing. Stair climbing machines require greater effort because you are lifting your body weight repeatedly.

Congratulations! Stair climbing is the final step. How soon you move from one exercise device to the next depends on you. An average progression is several weeks on each piece of equipment.

Walk Before You Jog

Performing lower-body rhythmic activity requires you to use your largest muscle groups in repetitive movements. Begin slowly and progress gradually. Walking for 30 minutes will prepare your muscles for jogging. When you can walk continuously for 30 minutes, you are ready to jog.

On your first walk-jog workout, walk for 7 minutes and then jog for 3. Jog at a fast walking pace. Repeat this 3 times for a total of 30 minutes. When you feel ready, walk for 5 minutes and then jog for 5. In a few months you may be able to jog the entire 30 minutes.

Jog in an upright position, stomach in, strike with the heel and then roll to the toe, taking short, smooth strides. Pick up your feet, lifting your front knee, and extending your back leg. Keep your elbows bent, your forearms and chin parallel to the ground. Breathe deeply from your diaphragm. If you feel winded, slow to a walk. Don't ignore discomfort in your shins, knees, or back. Pay attention to your body.

In Other Words

Static stretching means to hold your stretch. Hold your stretch for 15 to 30 seconds to combat the stretch reflex. The stretch reflex is a rubber band–like tendency that happens to your muscle when you stretch it beyond resting length. Your muscles want to bounce back.

Stretching Your Buns and Thighs

For safety, never stretch a cold muscle. Have you noticed that on warm days you can touch your toes, but on cooler days you barely reach your knees? That you can hold your stretch more comfortably in the afternoon than in the morning?

Go for comfort. Settle into your pose. Warm up for 5-8 minutes before stretching to avoid injuries. Exhale as you move into each position. Learn to hold your stretch for at least 10 seconds in order to fully relax the muscle. Add 2 seconds a week until you work up to 30 seconds. You may stretch to a slight level of tension, but never approaching pain.

Figure-4 Stretch

The Figure-4 Stretch lengthens your buns and outer thigh muscles. Keep your back straight and your head on the floor. Your neck should remain relaxed. Move slowly through your stretch. Stretch to the point of tension, never discomfort. Relax into your stretch.

After a few months, in order to stretch even farther, use your hands to pull your leg slowly toward your chest. When you feel tension stop, and then relax.

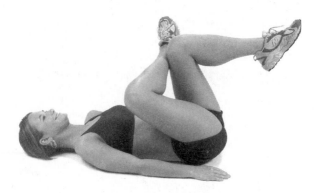

1. Lie on your back with your legs in a figure-4 position. Your right ankle is pressed to your left thigh.

2. Slowly draw your left thigh toward your chest.

3. Switch legs and repeat.

Straddle Stretch

The Straddle Stretch loosens your inner thighs and hamstrings. Lead with your chest, keep your head up, shoulders back, and relax. Walk your hands out in front and focus on your hamstrings and inner thighs. Keep your toes pointed up and do not allow your back to round. Hinge from your hip. Keep your back and knees straight. Exhale into your stretch.

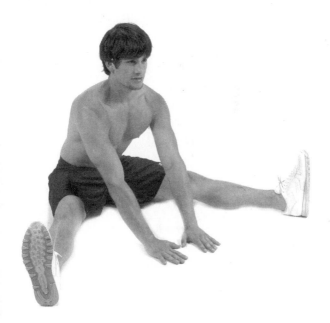

1. Sit with your legs spread out as far as comfortable.

2. Slowly lower your chest toward the floor.

3. When you feel tension, stop and hold.

Thigh Stretch

The Thigh Stretch lengthens the front of your upper leg. Maintain perfect posture and relax into the stretch. Resist the temptation to look down at your foot.

After a few months, attempt the stretch without using the wall for balance. A few months after that, if you feel comfortable, grab the top of your foot with your other hand. If you have knee problems, you may choose a different stretch.

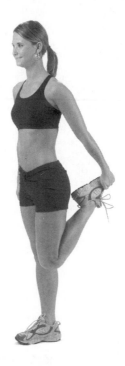

1. Stand with your right hand holding a wall for balance. Bend your left knee behind you

and grab the top of your left foot with your left hand. Exhale and hold.

2. Switch legs and repeat.

Side of Thigh Stretch

The Side of Thigh Stretch lengthens the muscle and tendon on the side of your upper thigh. Relax into your stretch until you feel light tension. This stretch improves with practice. It doesn't matter how far someone else can stretch, or what the model in the photo does. The more flexible you are, the farther you have to stretch. You may practice this stretch without a wall.

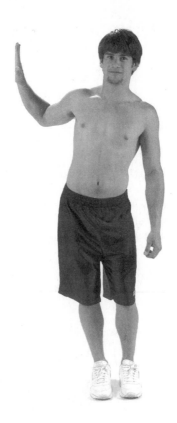

1. Stand with your feet together. Your right hip should be facing the wall. Place your right hand on the wall and lean your right hip toward the wall.

Butt Stretch

The butt stretch is very relaxing after sitting all day. Be aware that one hip may be more flexible than the other. Hinge from your hip and keep your back straight. Keep your shoulders down and your neck in line with your spine. Exhale and hold each stretch until you feel tension.

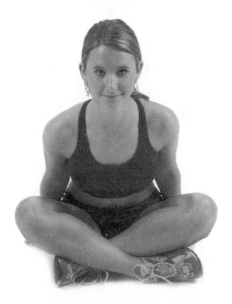

1. Sit with one leg crossed over the other and your knees bent.

2. Lean forward, leading with your chest until you feel a stretch in your buns.

3. Switch legs and repeat.

Chapter 8

Eat Smart

In This Chapter

- Cellulite be gone
- Don't eat the bun for sculpted buns
- Fill 'er up with high octane
- Sensible eating to lose
- Delicious, nutritious, will not make you fat

You may have tried one diet after another with no long-term success. You stopped eating carbohydrates and noticed a rapid weight loss. This looked and felt okay at first, but in a few short weeks, water weight returned and you still couldn't see your well-shaped buns under all of the flab.

You tried a low-carb diet but fell off the wagon. The same foods you abandoned when you started your diet were the ones that caused a binge. You thought it was your fault that you couldn't resist cravings. You blamed it on lack of willpower. But you didn't fail. Your diet failed.

A Diet You Can Live On

This program is not a quick fix where you lose weight fast and gain it back. There is no starving or deprivation. Eat cellulite-blasting foods—your favorite lean proteins, fruits, and vegetables. The program gets easier the longer you do it.

Rather than viewing nutrition changes as "going on a diet," make a lifestyle change or modify your existing nutrition plan to make it easier to maintain. Also keep a food journal to keep track of your nutritional intake. By keeping a food journal, you can also see what your body is responding to in a positive way or what is hindering you in your progress.

The program requires discipline, motivation, planning, and commitment. Get enough fresh air and sleep and minimize stress. Staying healthy makes losing those inches around your hips easier.

Picture a round plate cut into thirds. One third is a lean protein, one third is a fruit, and one third is a vegetable. Carbohydrates are an excellent source of energy for your leg workouts. Carbs get from your bloodstream to your leg muscles faster than protein or fat. Eat nutrient-dense fruits, veggies, and whole grains to fuel your muscles and starve the cellulite.

 Bet You Didn't Know _____

Any diet that restricts a certain food group won't work in the long term. Short-term diets yield short-term results.

Nutrient-dense carbs don't add inches to your hips and thighs; eating too many calories does. If you eat more than you burn, regardless of the source of those calories (carbohydrates, proteins, or fats), your buns turn to mush.

Carbs are good and protein is great. Eat a little protein at every meal. Proteins are your building blocks to firmer buns and toned, sleek thighs. Protein also makes you feel full longer so you are less likely to raid the fridge when you don't need to.

If you eat animal protein, choose the leaner cuts. Vegetarians can choose from tofu and the bean family to fulfill their protein requirement. Beans and peas are digested slowly so they provide you with long-term energy for your bun and thigh workouts.

Carbs and protein are necessary macronutrients to shape your buns and thighs. But don't forget about dietary fat. Dietary fat has received a bad rap because it has so many calories. Eat the right kind of dietary fat and you can't go wrong. If you enjoy dairy, eat moderate amounts of cheese and yogurt. A handful of nuts or seeds is a great way to get your essential fat. Eat fish several days a week. Use canola and flaxseed oil and stay away from trans fat.

Get It Right

Combine protein and carbs. Protein slow-releases the carbs into your system for better utilization of nutrients.

Eat to Fuel Your Muscles

Whatever goes around comes around when you eat too much. Make sure fat doesn't come around your thighs in the form of dreaded cellulite. Fat-laden, processed, and sugary foods will no longer provide extra cellulite for your hips and upper thighs.

Eat about 60 percent of your calories from nutrient-dense carbohydrates, 15 to 25 percent from lean protein, and less than 20 percent from essential fat.

It's almost impossible to drink too much water. Drink enough water so that your urine is clear, and that you feel a need to relieve yourself every two hours. Water helps to speed up the cellulite-burning process and aid your metabolism. Water is your first choice of liquid fuel, but until you take the plunge, drink flavored water and tea. Juices are 95 percent water, and soups, grapes, and yogurt are mostly water.

Eating Right All Day

Your blood sugar rises and falls depending on your activity, your metabolism, and how long you wait between meals. If you forego breakfast, have a salad for lunch, and then can't stop eating all night, short-circuit this chain of events by proper planning. Instead of saying, "I will never binge at night," propose a more realistic strategy: "I will eat throughout the day to prevent overeating at night." Schedule a reasonable after-dinner mini-meal instead of succumbing to an uncontrolled binge.

Eat a minimum of three meals a day to boost your metabolism. Use a variety of mid-meal snacks if you need to fill in the gaps. Munching frequent mini-meals insures that the food you eat is used for energy and muscle toning rather than for cellulite around your hips.

If reading this chapter makes you hungry, that is good. Hunger is a healthy sign. But there is a difference between being hungry and feeling famished. Know when you are hungry, and have the right fuel to feed your muscles. The best way to satisfy hunger is to eat. Eat before you get too hungry.

Fit your nutrition into your crammed schedule by keeping a ready supply of healthy snacks on hand. Prepare foods in advance. If you know you will be without food for a while, have healthy snacks available. Spend a few minutes each evening planning the next day's meals and snacks. Keep your desk drawer stocked with cereal bars, pretzels, dried fruit, dried soups, and oatmeal.

In Other Words

If you don't take in enough salt, you work out for hours at a time, and you drink too much water, you may become ill with water intoxication, a.k.a. hyponatremia.

Cellulite feeds off of processed, refined, man-made, calorically dense foods. You can't go wrong by eating God-given, close-to-the-ground fruits and veggies. Grapefruit, oranges, and other citrus fruits are among the best fruits. They're rich in potassium and vitamin C. An apple fills you up better than the same amount of calories from candy.

Your body digests and processes the food you eat, so there is a slight increase in your caloric expenditure during mealtime. It seems counterintuitive, but while you are chowing down, you are actually losing a little cellulite. If you already graze on five or six meals a day, don't stop.

Under-eating leads to cheating. Don't skip meals. Craving sweets may mean that you are not eating enough throughout the day.

It is better to be disciplined about your eating than fanatical. Choose round steak instead of hamburger; pork loin instead of bacon; baked potatoes, rice, and beans instead of French fries, fried rice, and refried beans.

Unlike tablet supplements, fruits and vegetables offer far more than just vitamins. They also contain fiber and other compounds that are essential to reducing unsightly cellulite around your hips and thighs. Feed your muscle and starve your fat. Eat and drink just enough to satisfy.

Eating for Your Workout

You may burn 300 to 500 calories during your workout. Therefore, be sure you eat enough to maintain your hard-earned muscle. You burn more cellulite if you work out harder. Don't follow the advice of anyone who tells you that you must train easy and slow in order to burn fat.

Your muscles love to be fed before and after the workout. Eating before your workout provides your muscles with ample energy. Eating after your workout revitalizes and refuels them.

After your workout, grab a sports drink or glass of juice to energize worn-out muscles. Your depleted muscles need energy to return to normal function. Consuming protein and carbs after a workout will also aid in repairing and rebuilding muscle, and replenish the glycogen stores you need. Look for a sports drink with between 10 and 20 grams of carbohydrates per 8-ounce serving. Your next workout will feel easier if you refuel your muscle as soon as you have completed that last set of squats.

The quantity of food that you eat before and after your workout depends on your metabolism and your activity. The harder the activity, the more calories you need. If you want to be scientific, eat at least 10 times your body weight in calories to maintain your hard-earned muscle. If you weigh 150 pounds, eat at least 1,500 calories throughout the day.

Eat to Starve Your Fat Cells

If you don't eat enough or you eat too much, you add more cellulite to your hips. Fuel your muscles but not your fat. Trial and error will help you to establish a balanced eating style based on foods that slim those thighs and are tasty.

As you develop defined lower-body muscles, you will be able to eat more food to fuel your increased muscle. Your friends will be wondering how you can eat so much and still maintain your incredible shape.

Eating perfectly all of the time is impossible. Any time you tell yourself you can't have something, you want it more. All of your favorite foods are part of your eating program. It's up to you to decide when and how much to treat yourself. During a weak moment, pinch the fat on your buns. Grab an inch of fat between your thumb and index finger and then decide if you really need to eat.

All of us cheat; some with greater regularity than others. A weekend cheat is the norm. Others need a cheat-food every other day. Or you may indulge in a cheat-treat every day. The number of cheat days, meals, and treats you can have depends on your activity level. A tape measure around your waist each month will help make your decision.

After a month on the program, hop on the scale. If you're losing weight, losing inches around your hips and thighs, and your legs are getting stronger, you're doing everything right. But if you're gaining weight and gaining inches around those hips, you need to adjust your cheat schedule.

Your Personal Trainer

A pocket spiral notebook will help you to determine if you are eating right or cheating too much.

Simply write down the foods you eat for a week. It may be tedious at first, but keeping a food diary requires you to pay attention to everything you eat. Keep track of when, what, and why you ate. Did you eat because you were hungry, bored, tired, or nervous? You don't have to keep a diary forever, but it is one of the best tools to get you those well-deserved buns.

Once you make your decision to eat clean, there is no going back. Not only is eating right good for reducing cellulite, but it is pleasurable. You feel energized and proud of your chiseled lower body. You'll know when you lose that extra fat simply because you'll feel better. You won't have trouble slipping on your jeans. Don't worry about the scale. Instead, focus on how your clothes fit. If your pants grow larger and your energy levels increase, you are on the program for life.

Your eating program is something that you do all of the time. It's not a diet you go on and off of. Eat several times a day to fuel your muscle and keep your metabolism revved. Drink lots of water—and you can't go wrong by eating fruits and veggies. A combination of whole grains, lean meat, and natural foods that are grown instead of made, will energize your muscle and starve your fat cells in a way of eating that you can maintain for the rest of your life.

Chapter 9

Doing It Right

In This Chapter

- Train your lower body every day
- Bun and thigh toners
- Rock-hard buns and thighs
- Putting it all together
- Eating and exercise = results

When it comes to firming your lower body, less is more. Getting great wheels is a combination of your diet, easy activity, and your favorite bun- and thigh-toning workouts.

Lack of firmness in the lower body is from excess fat rather than untrained muscle. Women especially may find that their inner thighs are a storage site for excess fat. To lose cellulite, doing hundreds of squats is not the answer. You lose fat all over, not in a single region from doing a specific exercise. The best exercise to reduce fat around your hips and thighs is easy activity.

You don't have to train hours a day to slim your hips. If you have several five-minute breaks throughout the day that's all you need. The best time to work out is when it fits your schedule. Do office hip and thigh toners every few minutes throughout the day. You can exercise while standing in line or sitting on a bus.

Doing part of the program will give you part of the results. Doing squats and lunges without paying attention to your eating and easy activity may grow your muscle, but you still won't be able to fit into your jeans. If you go on a diet but you don't exercise, you'll lose some cellulite, but you may also lose that rounded firm bottom if you don't include some toning exercises. Take a chance and try all three parts of the program for a month. You have nothing to lose but a chance to get great gams.

Do Rhythmic Training Five Days Per Week

Moving burns calories. Figure out ways not to sit on the couch. If you get up every time you change the channel, you are a few steps closer to sculpted buns and thighs. Stand up while you're talking on the phone. Better yet, pace back and forth.

Don't become overzealous about your workouts. Add activity into your life gradually. If you do too much too soon you will return to your sedentary life.

You Have to Move to Lose

You don't have to work up a sweat to slice off cellulite and show definition in your thighs. Fat burning can be as simple as stepping up and down while sitting at your computer. You could pedal a tiny bicycle underneath your desk, use a miniature step machine on your breaks, or simply walk around your office for 20 minutes. Whether you are watching TV or typing on your keyboard, remind yourself to get up and move every few minutes. Use your watch to calculate the duration of your workouts. Make a note of how many minutes you walk each day. Five minutes here, ten minutes there and your daily workout will add up to between 30 minutes to an hour. Shedding fat around your bottom is a cumulative effort.

Bet You Didn't Know

When you move fast you burn mostly carbs. When you move slowly you burn mostly fat. It doesn't matter whether you are burning carbs or fat at the moment. What matters is how many total calories you burn during your workout. The more intense your workout, the more calories you burn, the more fat you lose.

Add Two Minutes/Week Until You Reach 45 Minutes

Twenty minutes of extra activity is great for your health and wellness, but is also important if you want to see definition in your legs. But don't stop there. Add five minutes each week and you will get in better and better shape.

The more conditioned you become, the more fat you burn even when you are sitting. Those extra few minutes a day of exercise accumulate into thigh-chiseling results.

If you have a desk job, stretch the kinks out every ten minutes. Walk to the farthest water fountain. Sip enough water to give you an excuse to walk briskly to a restroom. Walk to lunch instead of driving. Be creative. Find ways to move instead of sitting, and your good-looking buns are just around the corner.

Move Fast or Move Slow—Just Move

Every workout is your workout. Don't let someone else bully you into his pace. And don't compete with others. Let your colleague brag about his 10K while you develop dynamite thighs.

There is no need to push beyond your comfort zone unless your goal is to compete. Your body doesn't care if you walk, jog, or run the mile, just do it.

Be graceful in any activity you choose. Rather than sputtering to reach a painful finish, enjoy each step of the way. As you get in better shape your body will tell you when it's time to pick up the pace. As long as you remember it's not a race, your body won't let you down.

You should be able to talk in complete sentences throughout the duration of your activity. If you are huffing and puffing and burning, slow down.

In Other Words

If you improve your VO2max. you burn more total calories even at rest. Your VO2max. is how much oxygen your muscles use per minute during exercise.

After your body gets used to moving slow, you are ready to kick it up a notch. Your body was meant to move and it loves the challenge.

But before you progress, be sure your shoes are perfect. It's a lot cheaper to buy a good pair of walking shoes than to pay the chiropractor later. Be sure that your shoes fit your walking style. You can buy shoes specifically designed for your gait. Find an expert to tell you whether you are a pronator or supinator.

Regardless of your particular walking style, keep your form as perfect as you can. Maintain your body alignment with your weight evenly distributed. Imagine a string pulling from the top of your head keeping your shoulders back and head up. Your elbows should remain at about 90 degrees and close to your body instead of flaring out. Place your thumb and index finger lightly together to keep your hands relaxed. Your foot-strike should impact your heel, and then roll to the ball of your foot and then push off of your toes.

If you are absorbed in your thoughts while you exercise, that's great. But if you move faster to a lively beat, then strap a Walkman or mp3 player to your belt or upper arm and you're good to go. If you are in a high-risk area, lower the volume in your headphones.

Take a break from reading for a moment. Stand up and walk slowly across the room. Then walk back briskly and check if you are breathing a little heavier and if your heart rate increased.

After your brisk walk is over, you continue to burn extra calories even after you sit down. The faster and farther you walk, the more calories you burn for several minutes after your workout is completed.

Change up your program to get you to the next level. Begin with easy movement, and then gradually increase the intensity. Moving fast simply means moving at a pace that is challenging but doable. If you dislike cardio workouts on the machines at the gym, bring a magazine or book you are interested in to pass the time.

Warm Up Before and Cool Down After Your Activity

Program 1: Introduce intervals gradually into your steady-state program. While you are walking, choose a target up ahead, and walk a little faster until you get there. Then slow down a bit. When you catch your breath, find another landmark. You will be amazed at how quickly you cross your workout finish line.

Program 2: During Week One, move for 25 minutes, alternating 2-minute intervals of moving fast and 2-minute intervals moving slow. During Week Two, move for 30 minutes doing a 2-minute fast interval and a 1-minute slow interval.

Program 3: Move at about 60 percent of your maximum effort for 5 minutes. Take a 1-minute easy-moving break. Do this for 5 cycles.

If you hate intervals, don't do them. They are great to change up your program, but if you prefer steady, brisk activity, keep doing that.

Whether you're walking, pedaling, gardening, inline skating, swimming, or stepping, do an activity you love. The exercise you choose should be enjoyable, and most importantly, fit easily into your schedule.

Bun and Thigh Isolation Training

You can perform your isolation training at home, in your office, or in the gym. Train your legs no more than twice a week. Your leg exercises should take no longer than a few minutes. How hard you train your legs is more important than how long. Go for "the burn" occasionally, but if your leg muscles feel uncomfortable for a couple of days afterward, you went too far.

A red flag is joint pain or extreme muscle fatigue. Take a few days to recover, and ease back into your activity. If you feel pain the next time you work out, see your doctor and try a different activity.

 Your Personal Trainer

Never work out a sore muscle. Your muscles need to repair themselves during your rest days. If they don't get enough rest they will constantly be in a broken-down state.

Chair Circuit

If you find yourself in a seated position and you only have a few minutes to train your buns and thighs, try this quick 15-second bun-toning circuit. Move from one exercise to the next as quickly as possible. Hold each position for 5 seconds.

Press your heels into the floor until you feel your thighs, buns, and hamstrings contract. Then, without resting, squeeze your knees together and flex the muscles of your inner thighs. One more exercise—press the outside of your knees against your hands. Your outer hip and thigh muscles flex for 5 seconds.

In 15 seconds you worked all of your upper-leg muscles. If you have more time, simply do another circuit of the same routine. Three cycles would be perfect.

Perform 3 bun and thigh toners 3 times a week. Target each muscle with a specific exercise. Do 3 exercises per workout—one for your thighs, one for your hamstrings, and one that targets all of your upper-leg muscles simultaneously.

Mix and match. Your legs love to be challenged from different angles and intensities. Use perfect form to maximize your progress and minimize soreness.

Standing Circuit

If you are extremely short on time, but you are at home or in the gym, put the bun and thigh isolation exercises together into a standing circuit workout. The standing circuit keeps your heart rate up so that you get your legs toned and lose cellulite simultaneously.

Stand with your feet shoulder-width apart and do a set of 10 perfect squats. Then, without any rest, do a set of 10 dead lifts. Finally, one more quick set of 10 squats. By now you might need a breather so take a 30-second break and a sip of water. Then perform a set of 10 lunges with your right leg forward. Switch to a left leg–forward position and perform 10 lunges.

And there you have it—a cellulite-sucking workout in less than 2 minutes, and that included your 30-second break.

Each Week Add Two Reps to Your Program

When you first begin training your legs, they respond to almost any exercise you do. But if you don't continue to challenge them, they stay the same. That is why you should add two repetitions per week to your bun and thigh toning program. Look for visible results in a few weeks.

Add One New Isolation Exercise Each Month

Just as you get bored doing the same exercises day after day, your legs do, too. When you don't add anything new to your bun and thigh isolation program don't expect to see improvement. Adding one new exercise each month will ignite your progress.

Get It Right

Most people think lactic acid is "the burn" you feel in your muscles during your workout. The burn is actually caused by hydrogen ions that increase the acidity in your blood.

Eating Program

In the nineteenth century the Graham Diet was popular. Sylvester Graham, inventor of Graham crackers, suggested that if you eat a bland diet you will lose weight. His theory was that if you eat only bland foods based mainly on whole wheat without meat, you won't eat much, and you will lose weight.

Fortunately you weren't living in the early 1900s, or you might have tried the tapeworm diet to lose those extra inches around your hips.

The point is, diets don't work. If you cannot stick with an eating program for the rest of your life, it's not worth trying for a meal.

Eat a balanced breakfast every morning.

Most people overeat. Even if you eat healthy foods, you can still eat too much. Eating a substantial breakfast is the most important thing you can do so that you eat less the rest of the day. Your body stores extra fuel as energy in your muscles, energy in your liver, or cellulite around your legs.

Eat a protein/carbohydrate snack after your workout.

Eating foods that are rocket fuel to your thigh muscles goes a long way to reducing cellulite. Lean protein is necessary for the growth and repair of your brand new butt. Fruits and veggies contain vitamins, minerals, and fiber, which is important in losing the fat on your hips. Fiber helps you feel full sooner so you eat less. Also, fruits and veggies are low in calories and less likely to be converted into cellulite.

Below is a sampling of some foods for your eating program. There are hundreds more to choose from depending on your taste.

Sample Foods On the Eating Program

	Lean Protein	Complex Carbs	Fruit
❏	Eggs	Bean family	Apples
❏	Chicken	Potato family	Grapes
❏	Lean beef	Rice family	Oranges

Drink water before, during, and after your workout.

The blood is 82 percent water. The brain is 76 percent water. Lungs are 90 percent water. Losing as little as two percent of your body's water will hurt your leg workouts.

Drink about 1 milliliter of water per calorie that you burn. That means if you burn 2,000 calories working out, you need to drink an additional 2 liters of water.

Your muscles are most receptive to reloading energy in a 15- to 30-minute window immediately following exercise. The blood flow to your muscles is improved right after your workout.

Essential, Omega-Three Fats

Eating fat creates a feeling of fullness. If you eliminate fat from your diet you may tend to feel hungry and continue to eat additional carbs and protein. Too many carbs and protein calories add up to patches of cellulite surrounding your thighs. Choose products that contain omega-three fats. Foods containing omega-threes include fish, nuts, flaxseed oil, and canola oil. Limit your intake of saturated fat and avoid trans fat.

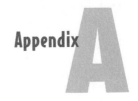

Reading, Viewing, Surfing

To get the latest fitness and motivation tips, check out some of the magazines, DVD/videos, and websites below.

Information in the fitness world is constantly changing, so it's a good idea to keep up with what's going on. You can also learn ways to spice up your workouts and add new recipes to your eating program.

Magazines to Motivate Your Buns and Thigh Training

Fitness magazine

Shape magazine

Self magazine

Men's Fitness magazine

Ms. Fitness magazine

Videos to Change Up Your Buns and Thigh Routine

Leslie Sansone's Short Cuts Lower Body

Janis Saffell's Brand New Butt & More

The Firm: Lower Body Sculpt I

The Firm: Sculpted Buns, Hips & Thighs

The Firm: Lower Body Split

Karen Voight's Lean Legs and Buns

Websites to Bolster Your Workout

Nutrition Navigator
www.navigator.tufts.edu.com

Gatorade Sports Science Institute
www.gssiweb.org

IDEA: The Health and Fitness Source
www.ideafit.com

Fitness World
www.fitnessworld.com

Calorie Control Council
www.caloriecontrol.org

Tom Seabourne's website
www.tomseabourne.com

Index

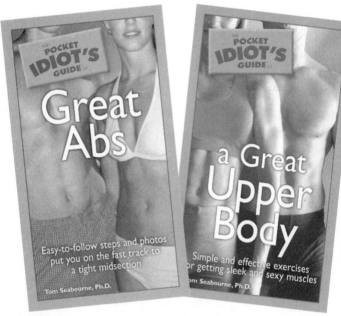